HANDBOOK OF
Good Psychiatric Management
for **Adolescents**
With
Borderline
Personality Disorder

HANDBOOK OF
Good Psychiatric Management
for **Adolescents**
With
Borderline
Personality Disorder

Edited by

Lois W. Choi-Kain, M.D., M.Ed.

Carla Sharp, Ph.D.

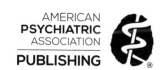

AMERICAN
PSYCHIATRIC
ASSOCIATION
PUBLISHING

If you wish to buy 50 or more copies of the same title, please go to www.appi.org/specialdiscounts for more information.

Copyright © 2022 American Psychiatric Association Publishing

ALL RIGHTS RESERVED

First Edition

Manufactured in the United States of America on acid-free paper

25 24 23 22 21   5 4 3 2 1

American Psychiatric Association Publishing
800 Maine Avenue SW
Suite 900
Washington, DC 20024-2812
www.appi.org

Library of Congress Cataloging-in-Publication Data

Names: Choi-Kain, Lois W., editor. | Sharp, Carla, editor. | American Psychiatric Association Publishing, issuing body.

Title: Handbook of good psychiatric management for adolescents with borderline personality disorder / edited by Lois W. Choi-Kain, Carla Sharp.

Description: First edition. | Washington, DC : American Psychiatric Association Publishing, [2021] | Includes bibliographical references and index.

Identifiers: LCCN 2021013695 (print) | LCCN 2021013696 (ebook) | ISBN 9781615373932 (paperback ; alk. paper) | ISBN 9781615373949 (ebook)

Subjects: MESH: Borderline Personality Disorder—therapy | Borderline Personality Disorder—diagnosis | Early Medical Intervention | Early Diagnosis | Family Relations—psychology | Adolescent

Classification: LCC RC569.5.B67 (print) | LCC RC569.5.B67 (ebook) | NLM WM 190.5.B5 | DDC 616.85/852—dc23

LC record available at https://lccn.loc.gov/2021013695

LC ebook record available at https://lccn.loc.gov/2021013696

British Library Cataloguing in Publication Data

A CIP record is available from the British Library.

Contents

Contributors

Marcelo Brañas, M.D.
Medical Supervisor, Adolescent BPD Outpatient Clinic, Department of Psychiatry, University of São Paulo, São Paulo, Brazil

Teresa Carreño, M.D.
Voluntary Assistant Professor, Department of Psychiatry and Behavioral Sciences, University of Miami Miller School of Medicine, Miami, Florida

Lois W. Choi-Kain, M.D., M.Ed., DFAPA
Assistant Professor of Psychiatry, Harvard Medical School; Director, Gunderson Personality Disorders Institute, McLean Hospital, Belmont, Massachusetts

Marcos Croci, M.D.
Medical Supervisor, Adolescent BPD Outpatient Clinic, Department of Psychiatry, University of São Paulo, São Paulo, Brazil

Carl Fleisher, M.D.
Assistant Clinical Professor, Department of Psychiatry and Biobehavioral Sciences, University of California Los Angeles, Los Angeles, California

Gabrielle Ilagan, B.A.
Lab Manager, Gunderson Personality Disorders Institute, McLean Hospital, Belmont, Massachusetts

Eduardo Martinho Jr., M.D., Ph.D.
Director, Adolescent BPD Outpatient Clinic, Department of Psychiatry, University of São Paulo, São Paulo, Brazil

Sara Rose Masland, Ph.D.
Assistant Professor of Psychological Science, Pomona College, Claremont, California

Carla Sharp, Ph.D.
Professor of Psychology, University of Houston; Interim Associate Dean for Faculty and Research, University of Houston; Director of the Developmental Psychopathology Lab and the UH-ADAPT Clinic, Houston, Texas

Disclosure of Interests

The following contributors to this book have indicated a financial interest in or other affiliation with a commercial supporter, a manufacturer of a commercial product, a provider of a commercial service, a nongovernmental organization, and/or a government agency, as listed below:

Lois W. Choi-Kain, M.D., M.Ed., DFAPA   *Royalties:* Springer

Marcos Croci, M.D.   *Royalties:* Editora Manole. Coeditor of *Clínica Psiquiátrica: Guia Prático*

The following contributors have indicated that they have no financial interests or other affiliations that represent or could appear to represent a competing interferes with their contributions to this book:

Marcelo Brañas, M.D.; Teresa Carreño, M.D.; Carl Fleisher, M.D.; Gabrielle Ilagan, B.A.; Eduardo Martinho Jr., M.D., Ph.D.; Sara Rose Masland, Ph.D.; Carla Sharp, Ph.D.

Acknowledgment

THIS BOOK IS DEDICATED
to Dr. Perry Hoffman, who was a catalyst for the recent surge in interest and action for early intervention and prevention of borderline personality disorder (BPD). In 2014, under the auspices of the National Education Alliance for Borderline Personality Disorder (NEABPD), Dr. Hoffman convened a group of about 25 clinical scientists working in the area of early intervention and prevention of BPD. At the time, this group of clinical scientists accounted for most of the individuals working in this area. With her characteristic energy and soft-spoken diplomacy, Dr. Hoffman, with the help of Andrew Chanen and Carla Sharp, inaugurated the Global Alliance for Prevention and Early Intervention for BPD (GAP). Over the past 6 years, GAP, now with more than 100 members worldwide, has significantly moved the needle in closing the knowledge-treatment gap for young people with BPD. However, much more work is still to be done, as most recently exemplified in a 2021 *Current Opinion in Psychology* special section, "Personality Pathology: Developmental Aspects." Several papers in this dedicated issue called for more generalist, easily accessible treatment approaches as an essential strategy to further close this gap. It is for this reason that we feel this book is best dedicated to Perry Hoffman, who first spearheaded the move toward this goal.

Dr. Hoffman was an exceptionally dedicated clinician, advocate, colleague, and friend to many. She was an innovator in bringing clinical professionals, researchers, patients, and family members together into conversation and collaboration to promote increased awareness about BPD. A master at promoting good teamwork, she was the engine behind the development of important resources such as NEABPD as well as Family Connections, which has grown to have an international reach and impact. Dr. Hoffman and John Gunderson coedited *Understanding and Treating Borderline Personality Disorder: A Guide for Professionals and Families* (published by American Psychiatric Publishing in 2005), an early effort to translate the latest developments in the field in an easy-to-comprehend manner as optimistic psychoeducation and guidance for both groups of caregivers. What was most extraordinary about Dr. Hoffman was her ability to identify needs, find resources, initiate movement, and nurture others in taking charge of what needed to be done. It is in that spirit that we remember her in our effort to help professionals start early in their good psychiatric practice for adolescents intervention of BPD, using the resources they have. Our efforts, like those of Dr. Hoffman, can improve lives, provide hope, and collectively bring about change in the field at large.

Preface

ADOLESCENTS WITH BORDERLINE
personality disorder (BPD) occupy a significant proportion of patients whom mental health professionals manage in psychiatric settings. From 11% to 22% of adolescents seeking mental health care in outpatient clinics and 33% to 49% of those in inpatient units already have symptoms that meet diagnostic criteria for the disorder (Chanen et al. 2004, 2008b; Ha et al. 2014; Levy et al. 1999). With enormous costs to those who suffer from the diagnosis, to their families, and to society, patients with BPD face major detriments to both their physical and mental health. Those with BPD represent a significant proportion of adolescents who self-harm and attempt or die by suicide (Marttunen et al. 1991; Nock et al. 2006). These youths encounter greater difficulties completing their education (Bagge et al. 2004; Trull et al. 1997), with ever-shrinking social and occupational opportunity, and ultimately are at high risk for unemployment and disability as adults (Winograd et al. 2008; Winsper et al. 2015). While facing these challenges, these adolescents have more troubled relationships with family and peers (Chanen et al. 2007), limiting their prospects for adequate support. The financial burdens associated with these complex outcomes are significant. A North American study estimated annual costs of $14,606 out-of-pocket and $45,573 billed to insurance associated with BPD symptoms in young adulthood (Goodman et al. 2011). When these direct medical costs are combined with indirect losses in productivity, the economic burden of personality disorders exceeds that of depression or anxiety, with overall costs of BPD ranking highest among these disorders (Soeteman et al. 2008).

These facts about BPD make the need for early intervention obvious. Patients with BPD should be able to assume that early detection and intervention are possible. Treatment for BPD should not be a last resort, initiated only once other routes are exhausted and symptoms become more severe and entrenched. However, a number of visible obstacles impede early intervention for BPD. Despite BPD's prevalence in psychiatric settings, overlap with other mental illnesses, risk for self-harm and suicidality, and help-seeking characteristics, sufficient training regarding its basic facts and clinical management is largely unavailable for mental health professionals treating adolescents. The sparse training that is available often centers on complex psychotherapies that are not scalable to meet public health needs (Chanen et al. 2020). The scarcity of general education about BPD in adolescence, combined with the intensive specialization of its evidence-based psychotherapies, contributes to the overall impression that its treatment involves a complex toolkit requiring substantial time, finances, and training to master.

Identified as "the disorder doctors fear most" (Cloud 2009; Shanks et al. 2011), BPD is a diagnosis riddled with stigma among health professionals. A number of common myths about the treatment of BPD in adolescents, outlined in Table 1, contribute to health professionals' active avoidance of providing early intervention. Even among those who are informed, out of a reluctance to stigmatize youths with the BPD diagnosis, some professionals sacrifice the opportunity to help patients and their families make sense of their many problems. Stigma, misinformation, and lack of training combine with the usual challenges of treating adolescents with interpersonal instability, emotional reactivity, and self-destructive tendencies to perpetuate the avoidance and lack of competence clinicians can experience in working with patients with BPD.

This handbook of good psychiatric management for adolescents (GPM-A) with BPD is written to overcome some of these obstacles by providing education and a general approach to the clinical management of adolescent patients with BPD. It dispels common myths that discourage treatment of BPD (see Table 1) and also provides a rationale to encourage early interventions using scientific evidence (Table 2). The education clinicians provide is meant to be shared with patients, their families, schools, clinical teams, and trainees as a resource for motivation in persevering with the difficult but worthwhile investments in treatment.

For clinicians who fear that diagnosis of BPD is pejorative and may cast a pessimistic shadow on their patients' futures, we hope you can be reassured that effective treatments rest on a balance between formulating symptomatic problems as pathology and broadening individual capacities to sustain well-being. New directions in BPD care call for treatments to achieve this balance by providing a sense of coherence that allows patients to make strides to good health by instilling "the wish…to cope (meaningfulness)," the belief that "the challenge is understood (comprehensibility)," and the belief that "resources to cope are available (manageability)" (Antonovsky 1996, p. 15; Fonagy et al. 2017). GPM aims to equip

---

TABLE 1. **Myths about treatment of borderline personality disorder (BPD)**

Myth	Myth buster
Personality disorders are enduring, inflexible, and pervasive.	Early in the course of BPD, some individuals experience symptoms as a single episode, and some with less severe symptoms move in and out of diagnosis.
Patients with BPD improve only if given extended, intensive expert treatment.	Extended, intensive expert treatment is required by only a subsample of patients; most evidence-based treatments for adolescents with BPD are time-limited to avoid interrupting usual developmental exposures that assist young people in building their lives.
All teenagers are "a bit borderline."	BPD symptoms decline over time. Adolescents who persist in having symptoms of BPD are identified for more focused intervention.
BPD is the product of abuse and maltreatment.	BPD results from an interaction between temperamental and neurobiological endowments in children and the caretaking environment with which they interact.
Patients with BPD resist treatment and angrily attack their treaters.	Difficulties may be symptoms of BPD rather than efforts to defeat treatment.
Recurrent risk of suicide burdens treaters with excessive responsibility and the ongoing risk of litigation.	Burdens of excessive responsibility and risk of litigation often are symptoms of failing treatments or defensive clinicians. Family involvement and discussion with colleagues can reduce clinician burnout and risk of litigation.

Source. Adapted from Gunderson and Links 2014.

---

patients to move beyond symptom management to management of life problems with greater resilience in the face of inherent sensitivities. This impetus places GPM at the forefront of new developments in the understanding of BPD beyond its traditional definition as a categorical disorder. Psychiatric nosology as represented in both the DSM and ICD-11 systems

TABLE 2. **Top 10 reasons for early intervention in borderline personality disorder (BPD)**

Reason to intervene	Intervention indicated
BPD in adolescence often co-occurs with other disorders such as obsessive-compulsive and avoidant personality disorders, anxiety, depression, and/or substance abuse (Loas et al. 2013; Winsper et al. 2020).	Prioritize BPD as the primary diagnosis when its presence will hinder remission or response to treatment for other disorders. Some acute comorbid disorders (e.g., SUDs, ADHD, manic episodes) often need to be prioritized, whereas others (e.g., panic disorder, MDD) will remit along with BPD.
BPD symptoms early in life predict other psychopathology later on. Adolescents with personality pathology have double the likelihood of developing anxiety, mood, or disruptive disorders, and SUDs in early adulthood (Johnson et al. 1999). Adolescent BPD severity also leads to steeper increases in SUD symptoms, which can, in turn, delay decreases in BPD symptoms (Bornovalova et al. 2018).	Prioritize BPD treatment earlier to promote better mental health outcomes by decreasing risk for developing other psychiatric disorders.
BPD features are one of the best predictors of continued NSSI throughout young adulthood (Glenn and Klonsky 2011; Wilcox et al. 2012).	Respond with supportive concern, help patients put their self-harm into the context of their larger life difficulties, and address the interpersonal precipitants.
The risk of suicide attempts is higher in adolescents with BPD, even compared with suicidal adolescents without BPD (Yen et al. 2013).	Promote productive coping skills, enhance the ability of trusted adults to support the adolescent, and instill hope.
BPD symptoms in adolescence predict a continuing need for services in adulthood (Winograd et al. 2008; Wright et al. 2016a).	Disclose the diagnosis earlier to decrease the likelihood of ineffective interventions and increase the likelihood of effective ones.

TABLE 2. Top 10 reasons for early intervention in borderline personality disorder (BPD) *(continued)*

Reason to intervene	Intervention indicated
Adolescents with BPD have poorer relationships with peers and family (Chanen et al. 2007). Impaired social functioning is associated with BPD symptoms such as affective instability, self-harm, and internalizing behaviors (Bagge et al. 2004). BPD symptoms have also been shown to have reciprocal effects on harsh parenting (Stepp et al. 2014b).	Engage families in treatment whenever possible. Provide psychoeducation about BPD symptoms, the interpersonal coherence model, and guidelines on how families can customize their home environment to aid the recovery and growth of their sensitive child.
Adolescent BPD symptoms predict school outcomes. As BPD symptoms develop, academic performance declines (Wright et al. 2016a). BPD symptoms predict not only lower academic achievement but also number of semesters on probation and ineligibility for reenrollment due to academic reasons (Bagge et al. 2004; Trull et al. 1997).	Work with school professionals to make a plan for reintegration and necessary accommodations and work with the adolescent on "thinking first."
Adolescent BPD symptoms are associated with a lower adult occupational attainment (Winograd et al. 2008; Winsper et al. 2015).	Focus treatment goals on functioning, or "getting a life." Teach the adolescent basic life skills.
Adolescents with BPD have poorer self-care (Chanen et al. 2007).	Provide psychoeducation on developing healthy lifestyle habits to facilitate better overall well-being and mental health.

TABLE 2.	Top 10 reasons for early intervention in borderline personality disorder (BPD) *(continued)*
Reason to intervene	**Intervention indicated**
BPD in adolescence is associated with significant financial burden. BPD symptoms in young adulthood are associated with estimated annual costs of $14,606 out-of-pocket and $45,573 billed to insurance (Goodman et al. 2011) and predict reliance on public welfare assistance for support in adulthood (Winograd et al. 2008).	Invest energies and resources for early intervention for BPD that can reduce future costs to individuals, their families, and society.

Note. MDD=major depressive disorder; NSSI=nonsuicidal self-injury; SUD=substance use disorder.

is moving toward a definition of personality pathology as problems in living related to management of self and interpersonal relationships. The time for a more generalist approach such as GPM is therefore right, especially in adolescence, when crystallization of pathologies into discrete disorders is uncommon (Chanen et al. 2016).

GPM is meant to be "good enough," to borrow a phrase coined by pediatrician and psychoanalyst Donald Winnicott (1953). Infants rely heavily on caregivers at first, but this must diminish over time in their growth. The less-than-perfect responsiveness of caregivers ushers in tolerable frustrations that eventually transform into differentiation of what a young person needs and what reality has to offer. This gap between the young person's need and what others provide propels ingenuity and adaptation as well as expectable frustrations, stumbles, and setbacks. We advise caregivers, including professionals, to be realistic and tempered, balancing attentiveness with allowances of independence. We also frame GPM as a path that has been charted by experience and research but expect that professionals, too, will diverge from its guidance and adjust its lessons. Explicitly, GPM was built through trial and error. It is meant to be practical, organizing, and predictable, but it will not always achieve desired results or solve every problem. We hope it will be good enough to aid efforts for BPD and its basic management to become widespread in mental health clinics and training sites.

Lois W. Choi-Kain, M.D., M.Ed.
Carla Sharp, Ph.D.

Chapter 1

Introduction to Good Psychiatric Management for Adolescents

Lois W. Choi-Kain, M.D., M.Ed., DFAPA
Carla Sharp, Ph.D.

The Need for GPM-A as Early Intervention

Patients with borderline personality disorder (BPD) should be able to assume that the professionals who treat them have been trained to do so. Equally, professionals should be able to assume that they will receive the training they need to provide good care for their patients. In this handbook, the authors present a basic prescription of what to do and what not to do in the care of adolescents with BPD. They provide guidance about how to provide such care, with usual components of good care for any psychiatric condition that most clinicians can readily learn or already know. After reading this handbook, you will have a basic updated fund of knowledge and clear framework for understanding BPD, which you can use to educate patients about the innate disposition underlying their vulnerabilities and to foster steady management of patients' lives so they can build mental health, self-esteem, and stability in relationships.

Every health professional will care for patients with BPD. The prevalence of BPD in adolescents matches or exceeds that of adults in both the community and mental health settings (Ha et al. 2014; Leung and Leung 2009; Zanarini et al. 2011). Symptoms of BPD first emerge during childhood or adolescence (Chanen and Kaess 2012; Chanen and Thompson 2019), typically increase after the onset of puberty, peak during early adulthood, and decline during subsequent decades (Cohen et al. 2005; Tackett et al. 2009). By age 16, 1.4% of adolescents in a prospective community-based longitudinal study met criteria for BPD, and the cumulative prevalence doubled during the remainder of adolescence into the early twenties (Johnson et al. 2008). Young people higher in BPD traits early in life are at increased risk for both retaining the diagnosis in adulthood (Crawford et al. 2001; Johnson et al. 2000; Stepp et al. 2014a) and developing other serious psychiatric problems (Winsper et al. 2020). Although BPD features rise and fall between childhood and adulthood, individuals who develop more significant personality dysfunction early in life are most likely to develop significant functional impairment academically, occupationally, and socially (Skodol et al. 2007; Winograd et al. 2008; Winsper et al. 2015; Wright et al. 2016a) regardless of the decline in symptoms. The progressive separation of young people with BPD symptoms from their peers and usual developmental trajectories precedes significant and ongoing disability in their adult years. Those who do not remit remain at risk for becoming more disabled and dependent on care systems as they become adults (Goodman et al. 2011; Grant et al. 2008; Skodol et al. 2002; Zanarini et al. 2009).

The opportunities for intervention are ample during this critical developmental period because adolescents with BPD, and their families, actively seek care. Patients with BPD constitute 11%–22% of adolescent outpatients (Chanen et al. 2004, 2008b) and 33%–49% of inpatients (Ha et al. 2014; Levy et al. 1999). Adolescents with both BPD traits and a BPD diagnosis are more likely to report histories of inpatient hospitalization and psychopharmacology, interventions with no proven efficacy in the treatment of BPD (Bleiberg 1989; Kaess et al. 2014), than previous psychotherapy (Bagge et al. 2005; Cailhol et al. 2013). BPD has also been shown to incrementally increase with other psychopathology in its association with suicidal outcomes (Sharp et al. 2012). Combined, this research has culminated in a call to action by the Global Alliance for the Prevention and Early Intervention for BPD, who declared adolescent BPD a novel public health problem (Chanen et al. 2017). Despite these advances, effective BPD care is often delayed for a variety of identifiable reasons, most prominent of which is the reluctance to diagnose BPD and its features early, as well as the dearth of widely available effective treatment options.

The Diagnostic and Statistical Manual of Mental Disorders, now in the fifth edition (DSM-5; American Psychiatric Association 2013) has included guidelines for diagnosing BPD prior to age 18 years since the third edition. Since then, research confirming BPD's prevalence, etiology, longitudinal course, phenomenology, differentiation from other diagnostic entities, and responsiveness to treatment in adolescence has converged with findings in the adult literature (for a review, see Chanen et al. 2017; Fonagy et al. 2015). Regardless, routine diagnostic assessment and disclosure of BPD in this age group have been the exception rather than the rule (Griffiths et al. 2011; Laurenssen et al. 2013). In the Netherlands, where national guidelines for early intervention have been established, more than half of psychologists acknowledged the validity of diagnosing personality disorder in adolescents, yet fewer than one-tenth reported doing so, and usually did so only in the context of the most severe cases (Laurenssen et al. 2013).

Discomfort with diagnosis of BPD in adolescence is likely compounded by the absence of treatment options. Although a number of evidence-based psychotherapies for BPD tested in adults have been adapted to treat adolescents (for a review, see Weiner et al. 2018), the small number of randomized controlled trials (RCTs) for these adaptations has not yet provided conclusive guidelines for treatment in this age group. The results of RCTs of BPD-specific psychotherapeutic interventions to date (see Appendix A, "Relation of Good Psychiatric Management for Adolescents to Other Evidence-Based Treatments for Adolescent Borderline Personality Disorder") show that BPD is treatable before age 18 years (Wong et al. 2020). Two of the most recognizable treatments for BPD, dialectical behavior therapy (DBT; Linehan et al. 1991) and mentalization-based treatment (MBT; Bateman and Fonagy 1999), have been successfully adapted to adolescent populations for the treatment of self-harm in randomized controlled trials (McCauley et al. 2018; Mehlum et al. 2014; Rossouw and Fonagy 2012). Both interventions show superiority in reducing self-harm during treatment compared with less intensive or usual care. In fact, DBT for adolescents (DBT-A) and MBT for adolescents (MBT-A) are among a few clinical interventions with positive findings and have the largest treatment effects for the treatment of deliberate self-injury (Hawton et al. 2015; Kothgassner et al. 2020; Ougrin et al. 2015). MBT-A yielded greater improvement in self-harm, depression, and BPD than treatment as usual (TAU) at the end of 1 year of treatment (Rossouw and Fonagy 2012).

Two large RCTs have compared DBT-A with enhanced usual care (EUC; Mehlum et al. 2014, 2016, 2019) or individual and group supportive therapy (IGST; McCauley et al. 2018). In both trials, DBT-A included weekly individual therapy, multifamily skills training, family sessions, and phone coaching. EUC offered once weekly nonmanualized treatment sessions. IGST is founded on the idea that "thwarted belongingness" is a risk factor for suicide, and, with individual and group sessions, it promotes acceptance, validation, and connectedness. Neither comparisons involved family to the same degree as DBT-A. In both trials, DBT-A yielded more significant reductions in self-harm and suicidality during the course of treatment. After treatment ended, the difference in outcomes between DBT-A and the supportive comparator became insignificant in the following 6 months (McCauley et al. 2018). In the trial comparing DBT-A with EUC, improvements in self-harm, suicidality, and depression were superior in DBT-A at 1-year follow-up but not at 3 years after treatment completion, except in terms of self-harm (Mehlum et al. 2016). At 3-year follow-up, patients in both groups sustained and continued to show decreases in suicidal ideation, hopelessness, BPD symptoms, and depressive symptoms, in addition to increases in global functioning (Mehlum et al. 2019). The findings in these major DBT-A trials suggest that both specialized intensive and usual or supportive interventions can yield significant clinical improvements over time, but more intensive DBT-A with greater family involvement may achieve these gains faster and with greater improvement in self-harm behaviors.

Finally, emotion regulation training (ERT), developed as an adolescent adaptation of Systems Training for Emotional Predictability and Problem Solving (STEPPS; Blum et al. 2008), is an evidence-based brief group therapy integrating DBT skills with basic cognitive-behavioral therapy that has been added onto TAU and compared with TAU without ERT in two RCTs (Schuppert et al. 2009, 2012). Both ERT plus TAU and TAU alone were associated with significant improvements in BPD symptom severity, general psychopathology, and quality of life, with no significant difference between groups (Schuppert et al. 2012).

A meta-analysis of seven RCTs of psychotherapies for adolescents with subclinical BPD symptoms concluded that specialized therapies provide greater improvements in self-harm and BPD symptoms in the short term relative to their comparators, but differences in outcome between treatment conditions were not found in follow-up (Wong et al. 2020). Furthermore, this meta-analysis found no differences in treatment retention or functional recovery between specialized psychotherapies and comparison treatments. Still, reduction in BPD symptoms across treatments in this small number of trials appears to be moderate to large in effect size, suggesting that both specialized and comparator treatments yield important clinical improvements. This meta-analysis was limited by the small sample and heterogeneous methods among trials, leaving implications unclear other than that a number of treatments for BPD and its symptoms are effective, without consistent advantages of intensive manualized BPD treatments over comparators.

Structured generalist early intervention appears to perform as well as manualized psychotherapeutic approaches. In Australia, Chanen et al. (2008a) conducted an RCT comparing the use of cognitive analytic therapy, a brief manualized psychotherapeutic approach combining object relations theory and cognitive therapy, with good clinical care (L. K. McCutcheon et al., unpublished observations, 2000), which provided structured, high-quality, general team-based psychiatric care within the same institution, focusing on problem solving, management of related concerns such as comorbid problems, and basic cognitive-behavioral strategies to increase awareness of dysfunctional thoughts as well as the connection between feelings, thoughts, and actions. Clinically significant improvement was attained in both groups, suggesting that early intervention is feasible and that good clinical care using general support and basic psychotherapeutic interventions was sufficient to foster clinical improvements.

Taken together, this first wave of research in the treatment of adolescents with BPD reflects three main findings. First, early intervention is feasible and effective in reducing symptoms. Second, intensive and specialized psychotherapies such as DBT-A and MBT-A may be superior in facilitating reductions in self-harm, but it is unclear whether the advantages of these treatments persist over time in comparison with less intensive usual treatment. Third, brief, structured, and well-specified generalist approaches to care can produce comparable and substantial clinical improvement.

It is unclear why more specialized intensive psychotherapeutic approaches that were found to be superior to usual treatment in adults have not also demonstrated clear and sustained superiority in adolescents. Considering the small number of rigorous trials and the abbreviated format of adaptations to adolescent populations, the lack of findings may be in part due to limitations in methodology (Jørgensen et al. 2020). Another plausible explanation is that adolescents may have distinct responses to the complexities of intensive psychotherapies originally designed for adult patients. The neurobiological, psychological, and social cognitive capacities of teens undergo tremendous transformations in the period between childhood and adulthood, necessitating modification of psychotherapeutic demands and expectations (Hazen et al. 2008). For example, the capacity for emotional differentiation appears to increase in childhood but decrease in adolescence, when developmental demands shift from identifying single emotions to differentiating mixed multiple emotions (Nook et al. 2018). Additionally, teens appear to be more sensitive than younger children to rejection (Rodman et al. 2017). The vulnerabilities of this developmental period put teens at risk for developing BPD and other mental illnesses (Kessler et al. 2012; Sharp and Wall 2018) and also may render complex psychological therapies more difficult to use, particularly in groups (Bo et al. 2020). Although important modifications have been made to evidence-based treatments for BPD in their application to adolescents, more adaptation and research may be needed to improve outcomes.

Informed rational guidelines for treatment are needed as the empirical validation of effective treatments for the age group continues to grow. For this reason, we adapted good psychiatric management (GPM; Gunderson and Links 2014) to offer good enough generalist care for emerging BPD in adolescent patients. GPM integrates early diagnosis and preliminary steps of intervention compatible with what most professionals provide in usual care. In this handbook, we provide a road map of basic interventions, including diagnostic disclosure, psychoeducation, management of self-destructive tendencies and emerging psychiatric comorbidities, multimodal treatment, and family involvement (Table 1–1). The book is meant as a practical guide rather than a technical manual that demands adherence. We hope this way of providing informed, structured clinical management enhances pragmatism, common sense, and a flexible attitude to promote what works to facilitate the natural course of improvement of BPD symptoms as well as functional abilities in the patient's life outside treatment.

John Gunderson wrote the original GPM handbook with an emphasis on what most professionals need to provide "good enough" care to most patients with BPD encountered in most clinical settings. As he wrote in the original handbook, "You don't need to be a specialist, to be selflessly devoted, or to have a larger-than-life personality to be 'good enough'; you need to be warm, reliable, interested, and unintimidated" (Gunderson and Links 2014, pp. 3–4). In developing this adaptation of GPM to provide early intervention for adolescents, we hoped it would provide a founda-

TABLE 1–1. **Distinctive characteristics of good psychiatric management**

Element	Distinctive features
Case management	Focus is on the patient's life outside therapy, not primarily on the patient's psychology as in psychotherapies.
Psychoeducation	Patients and families are informed of borderline personality disorder's genetic disposition, expectable changes, and the relative merits of different approaches.
Goals	Symptom reduction and self-control are secondary goals required to attain the primary goals of success in work and partnerships.
Multimodality	Psychopharmacological practices are integrated as adjunctive alongside endorsements for group therapies and family coaching.
Duration and intensity	No specific length and intensity are prescribed; patients and therapist collaborate in judging whether a therapy is effective.
Interpersonal hypersensitivity	An explicit and consistent effort is made to connect the patient's emotions and behaviors to interpersonal stressors.

Source. Reprinted from Gunderson JG, Links P: *Handbook of Good Psychiatric Management for Borderline Personality Disorder*, Washington, DC, 2014, p. 7. Copyright © 2014 American Psychiatric Publishing. Used with permission.

tion of wisdom and structure to steady clinicians in the face of expectable and usual challenges inherent in the treatment of BPD, with its hallmark self-destructive tendencies and interpersonal instabilities. It synthesizes long-standing clinical theory, modern evidence-based concepts, expert guidelines, and current scientific literature on BPD, specifically in adolescents, to facilitate and expedite learning for clinicians who will need guidance in usual clinical settings where adolescents with BPD will first encounter mental health services. GPM presents a reasonable introduction for patients and families to mental health care, using a medicalized framework to destigmatize the problems associated with BPD and focus treatment on minimizing symptoms, managing functional challenges, structuring expectations and roles in treatment, and promoting well-being and overall health.

GPM also offers a boiled-down introduction to managing BPD. Its ingredients can be applied in short-term acute settings such as emergency departments (Hong 2016, 2019) and inpatient units (Gunderson and Palmer 2019), as well as longer-term outpatient psychiatric clinics (Price 2019) and primary care settings (Adler et al. 2019). GPM maintains a flexible framework to accommodate any clinical setting, duration, and intensity of care. It embodies a practical case management approach that incorporates generic psychotherapeutic concepts and common factors found within most effective approaches across diagnoses. These common factors underlying basic psychotherapeutic changes include 1) instilling motivation that treatment can work, 2) building a therapeutic alliance, 3) promoting awareness of sources and mechanisms behind the patient's difficulties, 4) encouraging consistent reality testing, and 5) facilitating corrective experiences (Goldfried 2019). Although GPM incorporates these basic psychotherapeutic activities, it need not be thought of as an individual therapy. It is particularly suited for trainees.

Distinct to GPM is a central understanding that individuals with BPD are born with innate, partially neurobiological dispositions that make them sensitive to situational stressors (e.g., family environment, school), particularly to problems in relationships. This sensitivity feeds teens' sense of insecurity in relationships and in their growing sense of self in ways that destabilize their navigation toward a more independent life. In GPM, clinicians adopt skepticism about patients' inclination to grow permanent dependency on treatment or develop an identity based on being a patient. From a medical standpoint, it encourages clinicians to minimize harm first and emphasizes how surprisingly helpful treatment can be by avoiding common clinical maneuvers such as unguided polypharmacy and repeated hospitalization.

The Place of GPM-A in Treatment Planning

GPM-A is not an ambitious treatment approach. It strives to be generic and entry level, accessible to all patients and all health professionals. GPM eschews efforts to be superior, unique, or idealized, which can promote dependency and a sense of inferiority in patients with BPD when self-reliance and independence are developmentally preferred. GPM abides by realistic expectations that one can be adequate, well-intentioned, and reasonably informed but prone to limitations and flaws.

BPD's best-known evidence-based treatments for adults are lengthy and psychotherapeutically elaborate, but research suggests that intensity and duration do not determine outcome (Cristea et al. 2017) and that with intermittent, shorter-term, usual nonintensive treatments available in the community, individuals with BPD can improve (Bender et al. 2006; Paris 2013). In the treatment of adolescents, this attitude may prove even more important. Treatment should stabilize teens just enough to allow them to get back to important academic and social activities in their usual lives rather than provide a permanent haven from the demands at home and school that they need help learning to manage. As Gunderson noted in the original handbook (Gunderson and Links 2014, p. 4), GPM practitioners are provided this key mantra: "[L]ife's lessons can become a great ally in bringing about change if they become integrated. Treaters facilitate learning these lessons."

More specialized psychotherapies for BPD, such as MBT, DBT, and transference-focused psychotherapy for adolescents (TFP-A; Krischer et al. 2017; Normandin et al. 2015), continue to lead in innovating and testing approaches proven in adult patients for adolescents. GPM-A is not designed to compete with these treatments. These more intensive specialized approaches are for experts and treatment centers that have the interest in and resources to provide such care. These approaches are training- and time-intensive; therefore, they cannot meet the demand that exists for BPD treatment in adults (Iliakis et al. 2019). Their supply is even more restricted when it comes to care for adolescents. The mismatch between demand for and supply of BPD treatment perpetuates the tendency to delay diagnosis and BPD-focused care until a higher level of symptom severity and overall clinical complexity develops. For adolescents, this misses a critical opportunity for earlier intervention when problems are milder, less entrenched, and not yet influenced by the growing therapeutic nihilism that ineffective rounds of treatment generate in many patients, families, and clinicians. GPM-A aims to fill this gap by providing a lower level of less specialized care with some evidence from research that informed generalist adequate care can alter developmental trajectories of youths with BPD symptoms. Those who do not respond adequately to a general step of care or prefer specialist care and can access it should consider MBT-A or DBT-A, particularly when self-harm is significant enough to interrupt the patient's ability to remain functional and on a positive developmental trajectory.

As a first step in BPD care, GPM-A offers initial diagnosis and psychoeducation about the disorder, its expectable course, and its treatments. This basic orientation empowers patients and families to make informed and independent decisions about their own care. In addition, GPM-A socializes adolescents into the roles and goals inherent in a therapeutic relationship that does not always involve their parents. GPM-A encourages a supportive, relatable, and professional but human stance that invites adolescents to seek adult guidance, while also encouraging reasonable independent decision making and accountability. It introduces basic tools for managing safety and expects patients to ask for the help they may need. As noted, it incorporates common features of psychotherapeutic interventions for change, as well as common features of evidence-based treatments for BPD, including a structured framework; high levels of both patient and clinician activity; focus on emotional processing; attentive and nonreactive responses to self-destructive tendencies; attention to the treatment relationship, including relational ruptures and misunderstandings; encouragement of reflection and self-awareness based on a model of pathology; and the use of exploratory and change-oriented interventions (Bateman 2012; Gabbard 2007; Gunderson and Links 2014; Appendix A).

GPM-A also incorporates fundamental concepts of what works in DBT, MBT, and TFP in an introductory way that can pave the way to further work with those treatment approaches if needed or desired. When more specialized or intensive treatment is completed, GPM-A also offers a means of ongoing less intensive follow-up, occupying a role much like that of primary care for health maintenance, symptom management, and triage as needed. For patients, GPM-A is meant to serve a pragmatic role that is flexible to meet the situational demands of the patient's life at various developmental stages. For clinicians, GPM-A presents the opportunity to work from a generalist framework over the course of a patient's life span, even when BPD's most salient features may remit and its core vulnerabilities remain.

Stepped care approaches to allocation of different treatments for BPD have been proposed to optimize matches between clinical stage or severity and intensity of interventions (Chanen et al. 2016; Choi-Kain et al. 2016; Hutsebaut et al. 2019; Paris 2013). All of these proposed algorithms rationally match low dosing of treatment, more generic intervention, and briefer encounters with care for milder or earlier stages of illness. They outline steps of care that bridge identification of risk or early symptoms to further stages of illnesses, mitigating the polarized impulses toward diagnostic delay and therapeutic neglect or "premature diagnostic certainty and therapeutic overkill" (Chanen and Thompson 2015; Choi-Kain and Gunderson 2015, p. 263). To date, none of these stepped care systems have been tested empirically, and more research is needed to guide their use. However, they provide guidelines for clinicians to know when to apply which treatments depending on clinical circumstances. The limitations of stepped care approaches are that they assume that various forms of treatment are readily and sufficiently available and that patients' clinical presentations alone can determine match to treatment without assessment of patient interest, readiness, and motivation. General approaches such as GPM-A can serve a role at any clinical stage for patients where more intensive treatment is not indicated, available, or desired.

We would also like to note the relevance of GPM for recent innovations in the diagnostic classification of personality disorders, in particular the general severity criterion operationalized in Criterion A (level of personality functioning) in the alternative model for personality disorder (AMPD) in DSM-5 Section III (American Psychiatric Association 2013). Section II of DSM-5 currently preserves the tradition of previous editions of DSM and includes the 10 polythetic categorical personality disorder diagnoses that include BPD, categorically defined as a discrete disorder. In contrast, Criterion A in DSM-5 Section III requires an assessment of the level of severity impairment in personality functioning, defined as disturbed self (identity and self-direction) and interpersonal (empathy and intimacy) function. The new ICD-11 proposal mirrors the AMPD by including a general severity criterion as the entry criterion for diagnosing any personality disorder. Like Criterion A, the ICD-11 defines the general severity criterion as impairments in functioning of aspects of the self (e.g., identity, self-worth, capacity for self-direction) and/or problems in interpersonal functioning (e.g., developing and maintaining close and mutually satisfying relationships, understanding others' perspectives, managing conflict in relationships). It is critical to understand that the AMPD and ICD-11 define the general severity criterion as "the core" (American Psychiatric Association 2013, p. 762) of personality pathology and as being common to all manifestations of personality pathology, including BPD. Research (Sharp et al. 2015; Williams et al. 2018; Wright et al. 2016b) points to the possibility that the construct of BPD represents general personality dysfunction (Criterion A) due to the disorder's overlap with the general factor of personality pathology; its inherent severity; and, most importantly, the fact that its criteria reflect the intrinsic experience of maladaptive self and interpersonal function more so than any other personality disorder (Sharp 2018, 2020). The implication is that GPM is relevant for the treatment of all personality pathology not only because it was designed specifically in the context of BPD but, critically, because it focuses on general personality function regardless of traits. Put differently, GPM takes a pragmatic approach to restoring the capacity for "love and work" (compare Freud as quoted by Erikson 1950), or, in Gunderson's words, "getting a life." This is consistent with the ethos and meaning of Criterion

A, which assesses the degree of maladaptive self and interpersonal function as the core and common feature of all personality pathology.

Foundations of GPM

John Gunderson contributed to the establishment of BPD as a valid and reliable psychiatric diagnosis throughout his career as a researcher. His studies on defining BPD's phenomenology and features, formalizing diagnostic assessments, describing its longitudinal course, differentiating BPD from commonly co-occurring disorders, and evaluating its familiality and heritability provided the evolving scientific basis of his clinical management of patients with the disorder. Gunderson's first clinical guide to BPD was published in 1984, prior to the first wave of RCTs establishing manualized evidence-based care (Gunderson 1984). In it, Gunderson introduced a description of how symptoms of BPD fluctuated with relational shifts to important attachment figures, emphasizing an interpersonal focus in both clinical management and psychotherapeutic intervention. He outlined practical guidelines across therapeutic modalities and levels of care, encouraging simple supportive techniques and case management.

Clinical management directives of GPM stem from longitudinal research. With collaborators in the Collaborative Longitudinal Personality Disorders Study (CLPS; Gunderson et al. 2000), Gunderson reported that patients with BPD can experience enduring symptomatic remission in as little as 6 months without extended intensive evidence-based therapies (Gunderson et al. 2003). Longer-term follow-up in the study of BPD's naturalistic course shows that remission is likely in the vast majority of cases (Gunderson et al. 2011a; Zanarini et al. 2012). Interpersonal features (i.e., frantic efforts to avoid abandonment and an unstable relationship characterized by idealization and devaluation) were significantly predictive of the number of BPD symptoms persisting after 2 years, and the quality of relationships at baseline significantly predicted functioning after 2 years (Gunderson et al. 2006). The contribution of interpersonal factors in the maintenance of BPD symptoms observed in CLPS affirmed Gunderson's notion of interpersonal hypersensitivity as a central component of the disorder. Additionally, findings from CLPS on the interaction between BPD and common co-occurring disorders inform the GPM approach to organizing management of these disorders. For instance, the finding that BPD symptoms predict persistence of depressive symptoms in subsequent follow-up, but not vice versa, instructs GPM clinicians to treat BPD to facilitate remission from depression (Gunderson et al. 2004). In longitudinal studies (Gunderson et al. 2011a; Zanarini et al. 2012), functional recovery reflects a far less optimistic trend than remission; therefore, GPM addresses the need for patients to assume responsibilities in usual ways such at school and work to enhance functioning. Reduction of symptoms alone may not lead to increased functioning and is sometimes achieved in some cases in removing functional demands, which may continue to handicap patients with BPD in the long run.

GPM's guidance converges significantly with the American Psychiatric Association's (APA) *Practice Guideline for the Treatment of Patients With Borderline Personality Disorder* (American Psychiatric Association 2001). Although GPM can be practiced as an individual therapy, it centralizes case management as a more critical component. GPM's decreased emphasis on the necessity of individual therapy differentiates it from the APA's guideline out of recognition that patients can get better with brief, less intensive intervention and also the reality that psychotherapy often remains inaccessible at preliminary steps of care (Hermens et al. 2011).

GPM also uses concepts learned from more elegant and complex specialized psychotherapies such as TFP, DBT, and MBT (Table 1–2). Common to all these approaches is the imperative to think first, cultivating an interest in the way that interactions with others influence and are impacted by one's own emotions, actions, and understanding of events. This emphasis on interpersonal transactions overlaps significantly with both MBT's and TFP's focus on attachment and object relations. GPM incorporates the concept of splitting. As influenced by Otto Kernberg, GPM connects the way patients with BPD experience relational interactions in idealized and devalued terms, which come with associated anxious and angry emotional states. GPM encourages clinicians to make interpretations but does so in terms of the patient's predictable symptomatic abandonment fears and intolerance of aloneness. GPM instructs clinicians to manage boundaries and countertransference reactions by teaching them to anticipate urges to protect or rescue as well as reject or punish on the basis of these splits.

From MBT, GPM uses a not-knowing stance, encouraging clinicians to express their views as alternative perspectives while also providing empathic validation. GPM recommends healthy skepticism as an antidote to idealizing tendencies, promoting independent thinking as well as normal disagreement and self-assertion. These maneuvers also encourage realistic appraisal of the attribution of motives and intentions behind one's own actions and other people's actions, much like in MBT, but does so in candid direct conversation using an attitude of interest and curiosity.

Last, GPM embraces the notion that individuals with BPD may have social and psychological skills deficits that can be alleviated or managed

TABLE 1–2.   Good psychiatric management integration of prior evidence-based psychotherapies

Modality	Element
Transference-focused psychotherapy	
Concepts	Splitting and projection as defenses against anger
Therapeutic stance	Monitoring boundaries and countertransference
Interventions	Interpretation of anger; challenge avoidance and acting out
Dialectical behavior therapy	
Concepts	Social and psychological skill deficits
Therapeutic stance	Coaching
Interventions	Self-monitoring; homework; intersession availability
Mentalization-based treatment	
Concepts	Theory of mind; attachment
Therapeutic stance	Not-knowing
Interventions	Examining attributions about self and others

Source.   Reprinted from Gunderson JG, Links P: *Handbook of Good Psychiatric Management for Borderline Personality Disorder.* Washington, DC, American Psychiatric Publishing, 2014, p. 8. Copyright © 2014. Used with permission.

through social learning. Coaching, self-monitoring, homework, and some intersession availability are offered in GPM similar to DBT. GPM widely embraces what works and makes sense from other treatments in a sparing and focused way. GPM's eclecticism fosters integration with these specialized approaches if used as a step-up, a step-down, or an adjunctive modality (e.g., psychopharmacological management) to these more intensive interventions (Hersh 2019; Mercer et al. 2019; Unruh et al. 2019).

This current adaptation of GPM for early intervention with adolescents involves key adjustments (Table 1–3). First, because GPM-A focuses on both early diagnosis and intervention, it encourages identification of adolescents with three or more criteria of BPD (Chanen et al. 2009). With earlier intervention at less severe stages of illness, patients and families can benefit from identifying risks associated with BPD and will gain tools to manage symptoms, predictable difficulties, and risk more capably and with assistance. In this way, earlier intervention can decrease stress and increase support in the patient's environment. We have also fashioned many of the ready-made in-

---

TABLE 1–3. **Good psychiatric management (GPM)**
adaptation to early intervention

Key adjustments to adapting GPM to GPM for adolescents (GPM-A):

1. **Inclusion of adolescents with subthreshold BPD symptoms**—GPM-A's focus on interpersonal concerns and managing oneself is relevant to any adolescent with, or at risk for developing, psychiatric difficulties.

2. **Translation of materials into age-specific, relatable language**—The adolescent should be able to easily understand and relate to the treatment formulations.

3. **Family involvement**—The active participation of family members is essential not only in improving the family dynamics but also in keeping the adolescent engaged in treatment.

4. **Shortened treatment length**—Getting participants "back on track" as expeditiously as possible is recommended to avoid interrupting normative developmental experiences.

5. **Explicit focus on developmental concerns**—This is a critical time in adolescents' lives to work on identity formation, engagement in school, and increasing autonomy and quality of relationships.

---

terventions outlined in GPM to use age-specific relatable language to ease professionals' work in translating what we recommend into clear dialogue that makes sense to younger patients. GPM's inclusion of family in treatment is founded on the notion that patients with BPD are hypersensitive to important relationships, so their family will also need to understand the diagnosis. Family involvement is amplified in GPM-A because of increased interaction young people have with families when living at home. Although attention to family involvement is increased in GPM-A, it is balanced with a focus on helping teens build self-reliance and independence by managing symptoms effectively and building a satisfactory life that provides confidence to replace the insecurities inherent in the disorder.

Empirical Validation of GPM

Shelly McMain, Paul Links, and collaborators conducted one of the largest multisite RCTs of outpatient treatment for adults with BPD to date comparing DBT, the most well-studied evidence-based treatment for BPD in the field, with a structured, well-informed general psychiatric management approach to BPD over the course of 1 year of treatment and 2 years of follow-up (McMain et al. 2009, 2012). The unexpected outcome was that both approaches resulted in comparable improvements in self-harm, suicidality, BPD symptoms, symptom distress, depression, anger, and interpersonal functioning as well as significant reductions in utilization of health care (e.g., emergency department visits, inpatient hospitalization). Improvement in clinical features and treatment utilization continued and were sustained at 2-year follow up, again with no differences between DBT and GPM (McMain et al. 2012). Remission, defined as meeting fewer than two criteria of BPD for at least a year, was achieved in almost two-thirds of patients in both treatments by the end of 3 years.

The GPM approach used in the McMain et al. (2012) study, referred to as *general psychiatric management*, was developed by Paul Links, M.D., on the basis of Gunderson's *Borderline Personality Disorder: A Clinical Guide* (Gunderson and Links 2008) as well as the medication prescribing algorithm from the APA practice guideline for BPD (American Psychiatric Association 2001). In this study, GPM combined a psychodynamic psychotherapy approach with an informed psychiatric case management approach to BPD, offered in a weekly 1-hour outpatient appointment. The difference between this approach and DBT's 5-hour treatment package (i.e., 2-hour group session, 1-hour individual session, 2 hours of phone coaching) reflects not only significantly reduced treatment intensity in GPM but also broader generalizability to most clinical settings. The equivalence in outcome despite the difference in treatment intensity and dosing offers some evidence that effective treatment can work with less time, training, and specialization (see Appendix C, "Online Good Psychiatric Management Training," for a link to the GPM online training course).

In the trial of McMain and colleagues, GPM was delivered primarily by psychiatrists with interest and experience in working with patients with BPD. It was formatted as a year-long treatment, and adherence to its manual was assessed and maintained (Kolla et al. 2009; Appendix B, "General Psychiatric Management Adherence Scale"). Perhaps related to the active psychiatric management of comorbidities involved in GPM treatment, lower dropout rates were observed in GPM compared with DBT in patients with other psychiatric comorbidity (Wnuk et al. 2013). Another research group in Lausanne, Switzerland studied outcomes from application of GPM in a 10-session variant (Kramer et al. 2011, 2017a) that served as a starting point of care in their specialized psychotherapy clinic for personality disorders. They found in a sample of 85 patients significant changes in symptoms and interpersonal functioning, with medium effect sizes in their brief introductory variant (Kramer et al. 2014). Kramer and colleagues viewed this improvement as a remoralization effect that the initiation of treatment can provide when it helps patients understand their problems, establish goals, and build an alliance with a clinician. Adherence to GPM principles, using the rating scale developed in McMain's trial (Kolla et al. 2009), explained 23% of the variance in reduction of BPD symptoms and 16% of the variance in general symptom improvement in their 10-session GPM format (Kolly et al. 2016; Kramer et al. 2014).

Training for GPM involves just 8 hours in a 1-day course (see Appendix C for a link to the online course for GPM for adults) and effects important changes in clinicians' attitude and confidence in treating patients with BPD. In a study of almost 300 clinicians before and after this 8-hour course, ratings of avoidance, dislike, and hopelessness regarding the care of patients with BPD decreased, and feelings of competence, belief in their capacity to make positive differences, and belief that effective BPD treatments exist increased (Keuroghlian et al. 2016). Early career clinicians reported greater increases in feeling competent after the training than did more experienced clinicians. This may mean that less experienced clinicians learn in this training what many more established colleagues learn through experience.

A separate study assessed the same attitudes 6 months post-GPM training (Masland et al. 2018). Immediately after GPM training, clinicians again reported feeling more competent in treating patients with BPD, more willing to disclose the diagnosis of BPD, and more likely to believe effective treatments for BPD exist. Six months later, GPM-trained professionals reported increased willingness to disclose the diagnosis and take on new patients with BPD as well as decreased difficulty with empathy and decreased discomfort in treating patients with BPD. Considering that individuals with BPD are hypersensitive to others' attitudes toward them, these clinician-related changes likely influence the survival of treatment and the therapeutic alliance by increasing clinicians' optimism about BPD treatment.

When John Gunderson remanualized general psychiatric management for public use, he revised the title from "general" to "good" psychiatric management in the spirit of promoting principles of good care that helps clinicians think and make informed decisions rather than employ a technical manual requiring adherence (see Appendix B). Some essential differences between the *general* psychiatric management approach employed in the research study and the *good* psychiatric management approach presented in the handbook and adapted here include the following: First, the guidance provided here is presented with the intention to be flexible. Length and frequency should be adapted for each clinical environment, clinician, and patient. Use of GPM is encouraged if it is effective in helping patients reduce symptoms, facilitating BPD's natural course, and improving patient function. In the trial of McMain et al. (2012), general psychiatric management prioritized focus on self-destructive behaviors and emotional processing. GPM also encourages efforts to gain awareness and understanding of feeling states related to self-destructive tendencies but hypothesizes that those feeling states often arise in the context of interpersonal stress. GPM also places greater emphasis on functional concerns. Patients in McMain's trial achieved significant symptom reduction and BPD remission in the majority of cases; however, high levels of disability and functional impairment persisted (McMain et al. 2012). In response to this finding, this variant of GPM admonishes clinicians to attend to functional progress.

No RCT has studied this adaptation of GPM to adolescents. We hope there will be such a study to justify its use in the future. We hope that this book may facilitate empirical research using GPM-A. However, for now, we know that when it comes to the treatment of adolescents, general and usual treatments can help young patients be relieved from BPD symptoms, and an informed and structured approach appears to be good enough for most. GPM's equivalence to DBT in outcomes in adults suggests its potential efficacy in adolescents, and its overlapping contents with the good clinical care approach found to be as effective as cognitive analytic therapy (Chanen et al. 2008a) also suggests its suitability for a younger population. We hope that, for now, GPM-A provides a confidence-building approach for clinicians who want to follow guidelines for early diagnosis and intervention but need to learn a thoughtful and accessible way to do so.

Chapter 2

Overall Principles

Marcelo Brañas, M.D.

Eduardo Martinho Jr., M.D., Ph.D.

Marcos Croci, M.D.

Good Psychiatric Management Theory: Interpersonal Hypersensitivity

Clinicians, families, and patients often do not know how to understand the moment-to-moment shifts in the symptomatic states of patients with borderline personality disorder (BPD). Good psychiatric management (GPM) makes sense of BPD as a disorder of interpersonal hypersensitivity (Gunderson 2007; Gunderson and Lyons-Ruth 2008). Genetic vulnerability, endocrinological alterations, and neuroimaging findings suggest a biological vulnerability for BPD, which has been characterized as a stress-sensitive disorder (Crick et al. 2005; Fossati 2015; Kendler et al. 2011; Zanarini et al. 1990). BPD has a unifying latent genetic core (Distel et al. 2008; Gunderson et al. 2011b; Kendler et al. 2011), and interpersonal features are the most discriminating (Zanarini et al. 1990). The desire for exclusivity in relationships, insecure attachments, separation problems, and hypersensitivity predict adolescent BPD (Agrawal et al. 2004; Crick et al. 2005; Fossati 2015; Grant et al. 2008). These scientific findings suggest that individuals who develop BPD symptoms have innate predispositions for interpersonal hypersensitivity.

Normal adolescence is, by definition, interpersonally stressful, characterized by typical teenage dilemmas regarding dependency versus autonomy and individuation. Teenagers must navigate the intense challenge of learning how to manage different kinds of relationships (e.g., relationships with parents, teachers, peers, coaches, love interests) (Sharp et al. 2018) during a time when both brain structures and psychological capacities that contribute to "reading" or interpreting social interactions are undergoing vast development (Burnett et al. 2011; Choudhury et al. 2006). Adolescents must build a balance between exploring independence with all the usual risks and maintaining a bridge to the safety, guidance, and secure base of relationships with adults. The attachment functioning of teens becomes necessarily turbulent as social and emotional risks tend to intensify and the availability of dependency figures dilutes.

Intolerance of aloneness (Gunderson 1996) and attachment preoccupation, fearfulness, and disorganization (Agrawal et al. 2004; Choi-Kain et al. 2009) destabilize teens with BPD during this interpersonally complex developmental phase. The phenomenology of BPD changes dramatically in response to interpersonal context (Figure 2–1). Common interpersonal stressors can trigger abandonment fears, devaluation, self-injurious behaviors, suicide attempts, dissociation, and paranoid ideation. Splitting, or the tendency to see relationships in black-and-white terms, feeds into instabilities in how the teen with BPD regards their own self-worth as well as the trustworthiness of others. Interactions with others (e.g., parents, teachers, clinical professionals, peers, romantic partners) result in sudden and seemingly unexpected responses that reflect the mental states of being connected, threatened, or alone. When individuals with BPD feel "held" or connected, they can be compliant and agreeable, but they readily perceive rejection or hostility (Herpertz and Bertsch 2014). Any threat to that connection such as abandonment, criticism, or rejection, whether real or perceived, can elicit self-harm and angry devaluation of others.

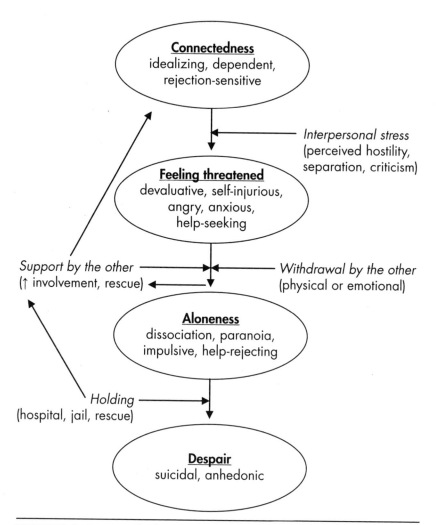

FIGURE 2–1.   Borderline personality disorder's interpersonal coherence.

Source.   Reprinted from Gunderson JG, Links P: *Handbook of Good Psychiatric Management for Borderline Personality Disorder.* Washington, DC, American Psychiatric Publishing, 2014, p. 14. Copyright © 2014 American Psychiatric Publishing. Used with permission.

When others respond in a soothing conciliatory manner, they might calm patients with BPD by assuring them that the relationship is intact. However, when others withdraw in fear or frustration, the teen with BPD can become more impulsive, paranoid, and difficult to engage. The absence of a containing relationship interacts with the adolescent's intolerance of aloneness and, during a moment of threat and pain, may give rise to a potentially more despairing suicidal state (Buitron et al. 2016; Hill et al. 2019; Kalpakci et al. 2014).

Stabilizing these reactions to being threatened and alone cannot depend solely on clinicians, or any exclusive, dependent relationship for that matter. Living in a stressful environment marked by unexpected separations or hostility can perpetuate a negative sense of self for individuals with BPD (Sekowski et al., in press). Paradoxically, some patients with BPD will cling to stressful relationships, despite their tendency to be destabilized by them. You can talk to such patients about how their actions may interfere with getting the responses they want from others. Patients can then consider more prosocial responses that lead to a more stable and supportive environment, which will in turn promote a more positive sense of self. You should explain that always depending on the likes of others (even you) for their well-being or self-worth is not a realistic plan. GPM for adolescents (GPM-A) aims to help teens feel confident in taking care of themselves so that they feel prepared and effective in the face of stressful challenges.

Using simple techniques discussed throughout this manual, clinicians can also help families reduce the stressfulness of their child's home environment and offer more stable scaffolding for the needs of their sensitive teen with BPD. By promoting the adolescent's sense of self-efficacy while also educating the adults around them about how to better understand their BPD symptoms, GPM-A clinicians aim to help patients stay on track developmentally. The goal of GPM-A is for treatment itself to become less essential over time as the patient becomes more resilient.

Good enough therapeutic relationships can provide a holding environment and foster a shift from a negative sense of self toward a sense of being good, lovable, worthy, and—most importantly—capable. Patients develop the belief that they are cared for and feel understood when treaters behave in a concerned, consistent, nonpunitive, and open-minded way. This positive sense of self can become internalized through a sustained and consistent partnership.

Basic GPM-A Approach

GPM-A holds eight basic principles that you can provide to guide the treatment of adolescents with BPD (Table 2–1).

TABLE 2–1. **Basic principles of good psychiatric management for adolescents**

Principle	Comments
1. Early diagnosis should be routine	A common mistake is to think BPD symptoms will be transient. Early detection is critical, and lowering the diagnostic threshold to three or more DSM-5 criteria is advised.
2. Provide psychoeducation	Share your knowledge about the symptoms, causes, course, and treatment of BPD with patients and families. Feel free to give advice when you feel it will be instructive. Keep in contact with the patient's school to help the patient resume and continue their job as a student.
3. Be active, not reactive	You are a role model for "thinking first" (i.e., not being reactive). Challenge silences, raise questions, use irreverence, and be curious (i.e., be active). Be active in talking about issues of concern to the patient's age group (e.g., social media use, sexuality, bullying).
4. Focus on life situations	Emphasize the value of school and structured vocational or extracurricular activities. Stay informed about the patient's relationships.
5. The therapeutic relationship is real (dyadic) as well as professional	Both aspects of the therapeutic relationship are essential. Acknowledge the ability to be supportive and also at times disappointing to the patient. Balance splitting tendencies toward idealization and devaluation by being careful to not play into them.
6. Convey that change is expected	Evaluate the treatment's efficacy and value if the patient is not improving. Collaboratively examine your contributions and those of the patient and family.
7. Foster accountability	While validating patients' emotions, hold patients responsible for their actions. Help them see that they can learn from mistakes.

TABLE 2–1.   Basic principles of good psychiatric management for adolescents (continued)

Principle	Comments
8. Ensure family involvement	Parents usually feel lost, desperate, and overwhelmed. Teach communication skills and how to manage crises. Build an alliance with them so they can play a helpful role in the treatment process.

Note.   BPD=borderline personality disorder.

Early Diagnosis Should Be Routine

A common mistake is to think that BPD symptoms will be transient when, actually, individuals who fulfill the criteria for the disorder in adolescence often may continue to show severe psychopathology in adulthood (Bernstein et al. 1993; Paris 2014). Therefore, early detection is critical. However, few early adolescents reach the diagnostic threshold for BPD, and subthreshold BPD teens have a degree of psychopathology and decreased health-related quality of life akin to that of teens with BPD (Kaess et al. 2017). Accordingly, lowering the diagnostic threshold to three or more DSM-5 criteria is advised (Chanen et al. 2008c). It is important to interview multiple informants, including the patient, family members, caretakers, and teachers, whenever possible.

Provide Psychoeducation

Sharing your knowledge about the symptoms, causes, course, and treatment of BPD is always a basic starting point with patients and families. Psychoeducation alone is effective in reducing BPD symptoms (Ridolfi et al. 2019; Zanarini and Frankenburg 2008; Zanarini et al. 2018). Developmentally, adolescents struggle to understand their emotions and how they influence interpersonal interactions as their social cognitive abilities mature. This is even more challenging for young people with BPD, who have difficulties in flexibly and realistically understanding themselves and others in social interactions (i.e., mentalizing;). Their dichotomous interpretations of events (i.e., splitting or black-and-white thinking) result in misunderstandings of interactions they have with others. To address these challenges, you should teach patients the interpersonal coherence model, the triggers and consequences of their symptoms, and how to better acknowledge and cope with these symptoms.

You will find many junctures where psychoeducation is a useful intervention, especially in your initial meetings with the patient, family, and other clinicians. Units and clinics can arrange psychoeducational workshops so family members can meet peers who share similar struggles. In many cases, it is vital to keep in contact with the adolescent's school. You can help teachers and staff working with your patient at school understand the disorder and its implications and discuss with them how to best adapt the curriculum and activities to the patient's current capabilities to facilitate a tenable life in school. Along with formal psychoeducation, patients can also benefit from wisdom about long-term life goals (e.g., vocational prospects, romantic life) and practical matters (e.g., organizing a calendar, techniques for studying). Emphasize the essential role that corrective experiences in school and at home may play in bringing more permanent stability to the adolescent's self-esteem and reactions to stressors. Support families and educators in their challenges and explain how the goal of treatment involves building a life outside the adolescent's status as a patient. (For a list of recommended online psychoeducational resources, see the "Psychoeducation" section in Chapter 3, "Making the Diagnosis and Providing Psychoeducation," and Appendix E, "Online Psychoeducation Resources.")

Be Active, Not Reactive

Patients need to feel that you are actively listening and care about their problems. Frequently, you are the "container" of the patient's projections. Adolescents with BPD often will exhibit different flavors of avoidance (e.g., passivity, disinterest, over-philosophizing). It can be especially difficult for them to talk openly about their feelings. They might say they are "fine," which in combination with nonverbal suggestions of the contrary, can be interpreted as Feelings I'm Not Expressing. You can challenge passivity when this occurs. Use humor and creativity when patients are disconnected from their feelings. If you are passive or quiet, this will be experienced as abandonment or hostility. Long and excessive silences are usually not welcomed by teens with BPD and are counterproductive (Zimmermann et al. 2020).

Be responsive, challenge silences, raise questions, use irreverence, and be curious. Do not overreact. You are a model of cautious and thoughtful behavior. Suicide, violence, and risk-taking behavior need careful examination, whereas overreacting (e.g.,by responding with hospitalizations, medication changes, or consultations) is often harmful. Taking unilateral action can work against the goal of empowering the adolescent to be involved in generating solutions to their own emotional problems. It is essential to contain ("hold") patients' projections and provide them with a model to be internalized. In order to do this, you can slow patients down, allow them to understand their sense of threat, clarify their feelings and wants, and develop thoughtful responses that are better received by others and less regrettable for themselves.

Focus on Life Situations

Because instability in primary relationships triggers BPD symptoms (e.g., anger, self-harm), it is important to know what is happening in patients' social environments, especially at home and at school. Work on their social perceptions and reactions, helping them identify the link between symptoms and interpersonal events. The goal is "making sense" of their feelings. Showing interest in patients' experience as legitimate and understandable is key, especially for adolescents. Advise patients on how to manage stressors and how to restructure relationships. Also, teach parents and other family members how to communicate more effectively with each other and make conciliatory agreements between their and the adolescent's values, needs, and desires. Guide caregivers in choosing which problems on which to focus their attention. Parents may need help to know how to avoid making too much of typical adolescent behaviors when there may be more relevant issues.

Adolescents with psychiatric difficulties struggle to perform well in school and have a higher rate of absenteeism and dropping out (Egger et al. 2003; Wood et al. 2012), which culminates in poor socioemotional outcomes (Gottfried 2014). Having structured activities can buffer interpersonal hypersensitivity by providing clear goals and roles, but adolescents will often focus on romantic relationships to the detriment of school activities and studying. Treaters should emphasize the message "school before dating." Helping patients identify their values and goals and how to build a life in accordance with them will foster resilience. You also should teach them how to better take care of their health and appearance; how to make sense of their free time; and how to deal with other important topics such as intimacy, sexuality, and social media. You can provide direction, but teens will have the job to choose what they do with your advice.

Most treatments for adolescents are time limited (see section "Setting the Framework" in Chapter 4, "Getting Started"). Excessively long and intense treatments can create dependencies that stall the teen's job of developing a life that fuels a more stable identity and self-esteem. You should gradually decrease the intensity of treatment, focusing on reintegration at school and real-life relationships. Booster sessions can be useful for keeping treatment gains.

The Therapeutic Relationship Is Real (Dyadic) as Well as Professional

You can teach teens how social interactions work by making selective disclosures (e.g., "You scared me," "That would make me angry"), acknowledging your mistakes (e.g., "I misunderstood," "I should have…"), actively addressing negative transference such as impatience and disdain (e.g., "Did I annoy/bother you?"), and talking respectfully and candidly. When considering to self-disclose, always think about what will help the patient (Table 2–2). Sharing your viewpoint can lend adolescent patients a position with which the patient can agree or disagree. This allows patients to clarify their opinions and practice skills of self-assertion and self-expression. Being overly afraid of making mistakes can rob both you and the patient of an essential humanizing process. The process of acknowledging and correcting your mistakes sends the message that relationships can be repaired. Idealization can be a positive sign at the beginning of treatment, indicating the establishment of a positive dependency. However, it is important to express skepticism of unrealistic expectations of you (and others) to help patients recognize the need for boundaries and limits because your relationship is also a professional one. You can teach patients a valuable lesson about how personal limits are important to the sustainability of reliable relationships.

Convey That Change Is Expected

Teens need to know that the usual course of BPD and its symptoms is one of gradual improvement, especially in the years ahead of them (Sharp et al. 2021; Winsper et al. 2015). Highlight that improvement depends on patients taking an active role in the treatment and that you are there to assist. Establish long-term goals (e.g., achieving satisfactory performance at school, becoming more skillful in social contexts). What the adolescent does in your work together matters. Patients should know that you have confidence they can develop better coping skills and that you expect progress. A lack of change is an indication of a treatment that is not working (see section "Assessing Progress" in Chapter 4). Collaboratively assess the effectiveness of the current treatment in terms of everyone's contri-

---

TABLE 2–2.   Self-disclosure by clinicians in treating adolescents with borderline personality disorder

---

Anonymity is a myth—for patients with borderline personality disorder, especially teenagers, it is fundamental to convey the impression that you are a real human being. Their ability to learn from you depends on it.

Ways that self-disclosure can help:

- Helps to mitigate trust issues
- Normalizes feelings and beliefs that patients feel shamed by
- Gives permission to feel, say, act
- Establishes authenticity
- Makes the clinician's advice more relatable and, therefore, relevant to the teen

---

bution (yours, the patient's, the family's, the school's), emphasizing that it makes sense to continue with the treatment only if it is working.

Foster Accountability

Underscore the importance of patients being active collaborators in treatment and in assuming control of their lives. Let them know that you will depend on them to tell you what kind of help they need. While validating their emotions, hold patients responsible for their actions and help them see that they can learn from mistakes to be more skillful in the future. Reinforce that when they can manage life on their own, their parents will not need to be involved as much. When setting limits, be clear about why. Do not impose limits in an automatic way. Evaluate collaboratively the impact of patients' behavior on their family, on their peers, and on you and whether or not their actions are effective in obtaining their goals. Equally, you need to be accountable for your own mistakes, feelings, or attitudes. Be ready to own them.

Let teens know what is expected of them during treatment (e.g., being on time at sessions, being proactive during discussions, trying the proposed tasks); ask what they expect from you; and tell them what you can offer, and what you cannot, in terms of your personal and professional limits. When telling patients what you expect from them, you convey optimism about the improvements that they can achieve during treatment, while realistically appreciating the challenges and mistakes that will inevitably occur along the way.

Ensure Family Involvement

Family involvement is vital, especially with adolescent patients with BPD (see Appendix D, "Guidelines for Families"). Parents usually feel lost, desperate, and overwhelmed. General and specific family interventions are available for BPD (see section "Family Interventions" in Chapter 7, "Multimodal Treatments"). Schedule appointments with family members routinely to refresh psychoeducation topics (e.g., interpersonal hypersensitivity) and assess their current difficulties. Parents need help providing space for their teenage child to grow their independence, especially when the teen's actions appear impulsive and self-destructive. Knowing how important their role is in so doing will help them contribute to the treatment's effectiveness. Teach strategies that can improve family communication (e.g., validation) and instruct the family on how to behave during crises (e.g., being responsive vs. being reactive, avoiding judgments, deferring discussion of low-priority issues until everyone is calmer). These measures will restore the family's sense that they can be helpful without taking control of the teen or the treatment. When the teen and family feel you are understanding and consistent, they will be more stable collaborators. Collaborate with parents on assessing treatment efficacy with an open and nondefensive demeanor. How treatment is working reflects not only on the clinician but also on the patient and parents, so these evaluations can facilitate joint problem solving to improve everyone's contribution.

How Change Occurs

Adolescents with BPD typically have a history of conflicts with parents, friends, and siblings (Skodol et al. 2002). In addition, BPD symptoms are associated with having more dating partners; placing romantic relationships above other priorities; and having higher levels of insecurity, intensity, and conflicts with partners (Penner et al. 2019; Reuter et al. 2015; Vanwoerden et al. 2019). Paradoxically, adolescents with BPD are more likely to date than their peers without BPD, but they spend more time alone (Kramer et al. 2017b). Early relationship intensity also may increase the risk of worsening BPD psychopathology (Lazarus et al. 2019). These findings reinforce the GPM-A maxim of "school before dating." This maxim is conveyed in a way that does not ban dating but encourages adolescents to prioritize more stabilizing components of their world prior to introducing more intense and complex relationships, which can be destabilizing for any teen, especially one who is interpersonally hypersensitive.

Clinicians in GPM-A behave and respond in ways essentially distinct from the adolescent's usual stormy relationships. They model candor, curiosity, limitations, tolerance of conflict, and dedication to resolving ruptures, which provide a corrective experience in the face of the patient's interpersonal hypersensitivity and fears of abandonment. These essential features of the GPM-A clinical stance render the clinician more approachable, relatable, and trustworthy to teens with BPD, motivating them to learn from rather than resist treatment. Therapeutic processes for helping teens with BPD are described in Table 2–3.

Learning to "Think First"

Teens with BPD usually are very impulsive, especially in stressful situations. Because of these patients' hypersensitivity, interpersonal events are the most important triggers for crises. Mistrust, insecure attachment, and regulatory deficits of orbital and prefrontal cortices over enhanced amygdala activation explain part of this phenomenon (Goodman et al. 2014; Orme et al. 2019). Under these circumstances, patients tend to overread or unrealistically assign complex feelings and judgments to others, confusing which thoughts, impressions, intentions, and desires are their own and which are of the other person (i.e., hypermentalizing; Sharp 2014). Teach adolescents with BPD to think before acting. Encourage coping tools such as chain analysis, introspection, writing, talking, and "counting to 10" to help patients delay acting on impulses (for a sample chain analysis, see Figure 4–2 in Chapter 4). The clinician serves as a model of "good enough" prudence and careful deliberation, encouraging the consideration of alternative interpretations when rigid and unrealistic certainty about others' feelings and motives arise (i.e., good mentalizing). Guiding teens to think first about the discrepancy between what they wanted and what happened instead helps them understand normal disappointment and hurt feelings, including the anger they may experience toward themselves and others. Putting this into context can diminish extreme misattributions to others as being neglectful or malicious or to the self as being bad or unworthy. Focusing on understanding how social interactions happen facilitates teens' ability to make better choices about how to respond to others effectively.

Social and Academic Rehabilitation

Adolescents with BPD usually are absorbed in matters related to interpersonal interactions, which are unstable and intense and precede crises. Clinicians have to convey an unwavering opinion that patients need to "get a life." Academic stability and family support decrease the intensity and

TABLE 2–3. Good psychiatric management's therapeutic processes

Process	Comments
1. Learning to "think first"	Under high arousal (e.g., social interactions), patients have more precarious deliberation—characterized by over-assignment of feelings and judgments to others, jumping to conclusions, and engaging in black-and-white thinking—and tend to act impulsively. Treaters must encourage, teach, and serve as a model of thinking before acting and considering alternative perspectives.
2. Social and academic rehabilitation	Adolescents with BPD usually are absorbed in strong negative feelings related to their hypersensitivity and difficulties in social interactions to the point where they are not able to function in school and other activities. Academic stability and family support booster self-esteem and emotional resilience. Consequently, adolescents are able to tolerate more challenging social interactions and find enduring partnerships.
3. Corrective experiences	You, as a reliable, responsible, and consistent clinician who acknowledges your own mistakes, serves as a model that confers security and can be internalized—that is, patients become able to soothe themselves. Feeling "held" and having practical pieces of advice on how to handle basic life situations improve patients' sense of being bad, allowing them to perceive themselves as lovable and more competent.

Note. BPD=borderline personality disorder.

frequency of crises. Schools may benefit from reading the "Guidelines for Families" (Appendix D) and adapting them to a school setting. After they are able to attain a stable and fulfilling routine at school and other activities, teenagers will be more resilient and feel better about themselves. Teens who are more resilient are equipped to manage more challenging social interactions and ultimately are more likely to find enduring part-nerships. Help patients recognize how their intolerance of criticism, dif-ficulties asking for help, and fears of failure cripple relationships. Remind families to "slow down" because their loved one has inherent sensitivities and progress requires time to be achieved.

You can tell families the following:

> We all ideally have seven layers of skin that provide cover, structure, and protection for our bodies. Teenagers in general, and especially those with BPD, have fewer layers of emotional skin and may be more easily hurt and disturbed. Teens with BPD may have only one to two layers of emotional skin, and the work of treatment is to help them grow more layers. Customizing the home environment to allow them space to manage successfully, with more time and scaffolding, will help them do that.

Advise the adolescent on how to gradually go back to school, perhaps taking a few classes at a time and choosing those in which failure is least likely. Set realistic and attainable goals collaboratively with teens and families. Teach them how to break down big problems into smaller com-ponents. Highlight accomplishments, but be moderate when making "you can do it" statements because they can be heard as you minimizing their difficulties. They also can—even unconsciously—equate getting better to being abandoned by you. The latter touches on an important point. Therapy becoming "obsolete" and ending treatment are welcome goals in GPM-A that you want to see patients achieve constructively. Ar-ranging booster sessions after treatment finishes can be useful for coun-teracting the fear of abandonment, making adjustments, and keeping treatment gains.

Corrective Experiences

You, as a reliable, responsible, and consistent clinician, serve as a transitional object who can hold the patient's emotional and interpersonal intensities by being responsive, rather than reactive, in comprehending their feelings (Gunderson 1996). The experiences of being understood and of trusting that you care about their well-being are often new to patients with BPD. These corrective experiences can foster a sense of security, founded on an interest in growing the patient's independence and self-reliance. When you acknowledge your mistakes and personal limitations and apologize, you convey the message that errors can be corrected and relationships can be repaired. Additionally, when you show that you are a real person, patients feel less intimidated to ask for help in a more direct way and to work on solutions to their problems with you collaboratively and actively. Through these interventions, you model behaviors that adolescents with BPD can learn, until they reach a point where they become capable of soothing themselves during moments of crises. These corrective experiences promote emotional resiliency and the capability for patients to be more comfortable with peers, get back to school, and perform better in their activities, which increases their sense of competency.

Chapter 3

Making the Diagnosis and Providing Psychoeducation

Gabrielle Ilagan, B.A.

Teresa Carreño, M.D.

Lois W. Choi-Kain, M.D., M.Ed., DFAPA

Disclosure of the Diagnosis

Adolescent patients with borderline personality disorder (BPD) often enter treatment for the first time, but rarely are they doing so with a diagnosis of BPD. They may not be seeking help at all and may be in your office simply at the request (or demand) of their caregivers. Teens and their parents may be in distress without a coherent understanding of the problems they are experiencing. Good psychiatric management (GPM) for any disorder relies on diagnostic assessment and disclosure as a means of making stressful and confusing problems understandable and therefore manageable. GPM for BPD provides a framework for understanding the stormy interactions patients have with those around them in terms of their interpersonal hypersensitivity, allowing the implications of this hypersensitivity to be discussed objectively and pragmatically. Patients have the best chances of positive outcomes when the diagnosis is made in an accurate and timely manner.

It is important to assess early symptoms that identify adolescents who may be developing BPD, including repetitive self-injury, impulsive risk-taking behaviors, both internalizing and externalizing problems, frequent anger outbursts and interpersonal problems, and insecurity in identity or self-esteem (Kaess et al. 2014). Co-occurring disorders such as ADHD and oppositional defiant disorder; negative emotionality; and temperamental traits such as poor self-control, low sociability, and shyness predict BPD symptoms. It is also possible that the BPD diagnosis will become apparent through observed interpersonal patterns that unfold in treatment (e.g., angry outbursts, distrust about your and the parents' intentions, frequent bids for your availability).

Disclosing the diagnosis early in the patient's treatment trajectory improves long-term outcomes. However, many clinicians hesitate to diagnose BPD, especially in adolescents (Laurenssen et al. 2013). A number of commonly held but inaccurate beliefs about diagnosis of BPD in adolescents have fueled this hesitation toward the diagnostic disclosure. These beliefs are outlined in Table 3–1, counterbalanced by up-to-date facts to encourage sharing observations about the early signs, risk factors, and diagnosis of BPD.

Diagnostic disclosure starts treatment with a clear focus in terms of goals, roles, and expectations. Knowing what to work on, who does what, and what the patient and family can expect provides predictability and direction that can be returned to in stressful situations. Contrary to claims that adolescents with BPD are simply experiencing normative teenage angst, BPD symptoms in youth are marked by their severity and pervasiveness and the presence of both internalizing and externalizing problems (Sharp and Fonagy 2015). Psychoeducation about BPD can also help differentiate clinically concerning problems from usual problems of adolescents, which can also be validated and normalized for both patients and their parents alike.

TABLE 3–1. **Reasons to disclose the borderline personality disorder (BPD) diagnosis**

Why clinicians do not disclose the diagnosis	Why clinicians should disclose the diagnosis
"I don't think the diagnosis of BPD is valid or reliable in adolescence."	• BPD diagnosis shows similar reliability and validity in adolescence as in adulthood (Chanen and McCutcheon 2013). • Diagnosis in adolescents is legitimized by DSM-5 and ICD-11 (American Psychiatric Association 2013; World Health Organization 2019).
"It's just teenage angst, typical in adolescents, that will naturally pass."	• Depending on the adolescent, BPD symptoms may remain stable, improve, or worsen over time (Wright et al. 2016a). • Even for those whose symptoms eventually improve, the presence of severe BPD symptoms in adolescence still predicts impairment in adulthood (Johnson et al. 2000; Skodol et al. 2007).
"The diagnosis conveys hopelessness."	• Disclosing the diagnosis facilitates the therapeutic alliance and hope (Shepherd et al. 2017; Sulzer et al. 2016).
"The patient will feel ashamed or criticized."	• Belief that the patient will feel ashamed or criticized is a countertransference projection that perpetuates stigma. Accurate diagnosis decreases stigma, blame, alienation, and anger and provides relief to patients and families (Pearce et al. 2017); S.R. Masland et al., manuscript in preparation, 2021). • There is no evidence that adolescents have a negative experience of diagnostic disclosure when delivered in the context of offering treatment, and adolescents receiving the BPD diagnosis find it accurate (Courtney and Makinen 2016).

TABLE 3–1.   **Reasons to disclose the borderline personality disorder (BPD) diagnosis** *(continued)*

Why clinicians do not disclose the diagnosis	Why clinicians should disclose the diagnosis
"I don't believe I can treat BPD."	• You do not need to be a BPD specialist to treat BPD effectively. • Generalist and brief approaches also effectively reduce BPD and other psychiatric symptoms for adolescents.
"I can help this patient without making the diagnosis."	• Sometimes this is true, but often it is not. • Disclosing the diagnosis establishes realistic expectations about course and treatment, prepares clinicians for their own countertransference, increases likelihood of interventions that work, decreases likelihood of ineffective interventions (e.g., polypharmacy), and minimizes interference with normal development.

Source.   Adapted from Gunderson and Links 2014.

The Diagnosis Anchors the Patient's and Clinician's Expectations

The BPD diagnosis equips the patient, family, and clinician with the knowledge that the patient has long-term vulnerabilities. Rather than casting pessimism, this message emphasizes the patient's potential to manage their sensitivity to stress, emotions, and social interactions proactively and realistically. It shapes expectations about the likelihood of symptomatic remission and functional recovery so that patients know they can get better but need to work to bolster their own functioning to build satisfactory lives. Provide information about both the effectiveness and limitations of medications to help the patient and family focus on what they can do to promote clinical progress outside sessions and treatment. In addition, psychoeducation about the course of BPD and other co-occurring diagnoses such as mood, anxiety, eating, and substance use disorders can frame expectations about what should be treated as a priority (see Chapter 6, "Pharmacotherapy and Comorbidity").

The BPD Diagnosis Fosters the Treatment Alliance

Disclosing the BPD diagnosis can provide meaningful context for the patient and family's difficulties. It creates a common ground for understanding the nature of these difficulties, decreasing blaming, and establishing a forum to address any maladaptive family dynamics. Receiving the diagnosis often reassures patients and families that they are not alone, that treatment can help, and that their treaters are knowledgeable about their problems on the basis of clinical experience and the scientific literature (see "Psychoeducation" section later in the chapter).

The Diagnosis Prepares Clinicians and Caregivers for What's Ahead

Knowing that your patient has BPD will equip you to anticipate their interpersonal sensitivity and help you understand when the patient will be more receptive or rejecting of what you have to say depending on whether they feel more connected or threatened. Without this framework, you might respond reflexively with caregiving or frustrated responses in a way that aggravates the patient's symptoms, so their capacity to collaborate remains unstable. Instead of responding to patients' dependency on and idealization of you with caregiving or responding to their devaluation with anger, you can help patients notice these tendencies and evaluate other ways of understanding interpersonal interactions.

Early Diagnosis Improves Long-Term Outcomes

BPD can interrupt developmental tasks for adolescents such as identity formation, engagement in school, building social networks and skills, and increasing autonomy. Identifying BPD early can help minimize BPD's interference with normal development. Medicalize the diagnosis to help adolescents understand these symptoms as something that they can manage and not something that defines them as a person. By treating BPD symptoms early, you may reduce the risk of persistent BPD symptoms, worsening mental health, and impairment in social and academic functioning (Greenfield et al. 2015; Wright et al. 2016a). You can sympathize with the stressful responsibility the patient bears to work on BPD-related problems to optimize health and functioning, while also making clear that these efforts can make a difference in the patient's immediate and longer-term future.

How to Disclose the Diagnosis

DSM-5 Criteria

A simple way to share the BPD diagnosis with the patient is to review the DSM-5 criteria for BPD (American Psychiatric Association 2013) together, relate these criteria to experiences they have shared or that you have observed, and ask for other examples of how the criteria may apply. This also has the advantage of involving patients in relating their symptoms to their personal struggles and unique problems. This collaborative review of criteria can set up the adolescent patient with BPD to have an active role in treatment and a collaborative dynamic with you to build your alliance. The patient is also more likely to react positively to the diagnosis when it is accompanied by appropriate psychoeducation and when the clinician conveys hope and optimism for recovery (Lester et al. 2020). Older adolescents may understand and identify with the DSM criteria as written, but for younger children it is helpful to translate these criteria into language they can relate to when needed. Suggested options for phrasing developed from structured assessments for BPD in youths are provided in Table 3–2.

Developmental Scripts

Depending on a patient's developmental age and family dynamics, the clinician may decide to disclose the diagnosis to the parents first, the adolescent first, or the family together. The following three scripts guiding disclosure involve the developmental perspective illustrated in Chapter 2, "Overall Principles," Figure 2–1.

TABLE 3–2. **DSM-5 criteria in adolescent-friendly language**

DSM-5 adult criterion	Statements the adolescent might share with you directly	Questions to pose if the information has not been offered
Frantic efforts to avoid real or imagined abandonment	"I worry that people I care about will leave and not come back."[a] "I have difficulty developing close relationships because people often abandon me."[b]	"Have you made desperate efforts to avoid feeling abandoned or being abandoned, such as repeatedly texting or calling someone to reassure yourself that they still care, begging them not to leave you, or repeatedly checking their social media pages?"[c]
Unstable and intense interpersonal relationships, with extremes between idealization and devaluation	"My relationships with people I care about have lots of ups and downs."[b]	"Have you often gone from loving and admiring someone to feeling that you can't stand them?"[d] "Do you get in fights with your friends a lot or have to take a lot of breaks from them?"
Markedly and persistently unstable self-image or sense of self	"I am often different with different people in different situations, so sometimes I am not sure who I am."[b]	"Have you often felt that you had no idea of who you are or that you have no identity?"[c]

TABLE 3–2. DSM-5 criteria in adolescent-friendly language *(continued)*

DSM-5 adult criterion	Statements the adolescent might share with you directly	Questions to pose if the information has not been offered
Impulsive behavior in two or more areas that are potentially self-damaging	"I get into trouble because I do things without thinking."[a] Specific behaviors: "I have often used drugs or alcohol to stop feeling what I was feeling." "I am often an emotional eater." "I sometimes buy things I don't need because it gets me out of feeling bad or empty for a little while." "I have often flirted/sexted/ been with someone else to try to fill a hole, to be wanted, or to get approval." "I have often stolen things when it wasn't on a dare."	
Recurrent suicidal behavior, gestures, threats, or self-harm	"When I'm upset, I typically do something to hurt myself."[e] "I have threatened to hurt myself in the past."[b]	"Have you tried to kill yourself?"
Affective instability due to a marked reactivity of mood	"My feelings are very strong. For instance, when I get mad, I get really, really mad. When I get happy, I get really, really happy."[a] "I often feel like I am on an emotional 'roller-coaster.'"[b]	"Have you often found that your mood has changed suddenly, for example, from feeling OK to feeling really sad or very angry or extremely nervous, fearful, or scared?"[d]
Chronic feelings of emptiness	"Sometimes I feel terribly empty inside."[e]	"Have you felt that you had no feelings inside? Or that there was nothing inside?"[d]

TABLE 3–2.   DSM-5 criteria in adolescent-friendly language *(continued)*

DSM-5 adult criterion	Statements the adolescent might share with you directly	Questions to pose if the information has not been offered
Inappropriate, intense anger or difficulty controlling anger	"I have little control over my anger."[e]	"Have you felt very angry a lot of the time?"[d] "Have you often felt really angry inside but managed to hide it so that other people didn't know about it?"[d]
Transient, stress-related paranoid ideation or severe dissociative symptoms	"Sometimes I feel like I am not real."[b]	"Have you often been distrustful of other people?"[c] "Have you frequently felt unreal or as if things around you were unreal?"[c] "Have you frequently felt as if you were physically separated from your feelings or as though you were viewing yourself from a distance?"[d] "Have you repeatedly had times when you felt spaced out or numb?"[d]

Note.   For clinical settings, the DSM-5 diagnostic criteria are sufficient, and advised to make the diagnosis. For research settings or if a more comprehensive assessment is intended, adolescent-specific instruments can be found in notes a–e.

[a]Borderline Personality Features Scale for Children (BPFSC) short form version (BPFSC-11;).
[b]Borderline Personality Questionnaire (BPQ; Poreh et al. 2006)
[c]McLean Screening Instrument for Borderline Personality Disorder (MSI-BPD; Noblin et al. 2014; Zanarini et al. 2003)
[d]Childhood Interview for Borderline Personality Disorder (CI-BPD; Zanarini 2003)
[e]Personality Assessment Inventory–Adolescent's Borderline Features Scale (PAI-A-BOR; Morey 2007; Venta et al. 2018)

After reviewing the BPD criteria with parents, the clinician can explain:

Some children are born genetically more sensitive than others. Their negative emotions are more intense, and they are more emotionally reactive. These children can be more difficult to understand and to raise. Their emotional needs can be unclear, and they can evoke intense feelings in their parents, making it more difficult to meet their emotional needs. It is a challenge to teach them how to self-soothe, and their hypersensitivity can cause many problems in their relationships. As teenagers they can be more intensely angry and critical of others, especially their parents, who have not been able to meet their emotional needs. They bring these desires, disappointments, and demands to other relationships, making it difficult to keep friends and to feel a sense of belonging. They can often evoke negative feelings in others and might be vulnerable to negative responses such as getting rejected and being bullied. They can also evoke guilty or protective feelings in others, causing rescuing responses that can sustain their unrealistically high expectations of having their needs met and keep this cycle going.

Older adolescents can likely understand the script for diagnostic disclosure designed for adults (adapted from Choi-Kain and Gunderson 2019, p. 15; Gunderson and Links 2014, pp. 23–24):

People with BPD are born with a genetic disposition to be highly sensitive and reactive to their caretakers. They are more apt to attribute rejection or anger to parental behaviors than are other children. They have usually grown up feeling that they were unfairly treated and that they did not get the attention or care they needed. They resent this, and, as young adults, they hope to establish a relationship with someone who can make up to them for what they feel is missing. The desired relationship is exclusive, setting in motion intense reactions to real or perceived slights, rejections, or separations. Predictably, both their unrealistic expectations and their intense reactions cause such relationships to fail. When this happens, people with BPD will feel rejected or abandoned, and they cannot resolve their anger about being treated unfairly and their fear that they are bad and deserved the rejection. Both conclusions can lead them to become self-destructive. Their anger about being mistreated or their shame about being bad or their self-destructive behaviors can evoke guilty or protective feelings in other people. Such guilt or rescuing responses from others validate the unrealistically negative perceptions of mistreatment of the person with BPD and sustain that person's unrealistically high expectations of having their needs met. Thus, the cycle is apt to repeat itself.

For younger adolescents, this explanation should be further simplified to be age-appropriate. For example:

> Some kids in your class are very tall, some are very short, and most are somewhere in between. It is not bad to be tall or short, and they were just born that way. In the same way, some kids are naturally not that sensitive, and some were born very sensitive. The kids who are very sensitive have intense feelings that other people might not understand. When they do not know how to handle their intense feelings and the people around them do not know how to help either, this can lead to problems at home and at school and can lead to even more intense feelings.

Psychoeducation

Although adolescents with BPD often enter treatment under urgent circumstances, it is important to take time to connect with them and their families to explain what the diagnosis means. Psychoeducation in and of itself has been shown to reduce symptomatology in adults with BPD (Ridolfi et al. 2019; Zanarini et al. 2018) and reduce subjective burden in caregivers (Pearce et al. 2017). It is also important in keeping the adolescent engaged in treatment. Positive perceptions of treatment by both the parents and the patient are among the strongest predictors of treatment retention (Desrosiers et al. 2015). Providing psychoeducation to both caregivers and the patient can help all family members prepare for the complications that often arise in the treatment of adolescents with BPD (Desrosiers et al. 2020; for other psychoeducation resources, see Appendix E, "Online Psychoeducation Resources").

Prevalence: "You Are Not Alone"

An estimated 1%–3% of adolescents have BPD (Johnson et al. 2008; Zanarini et al. 2011). Clinicians can tell their patients, "There are many combinations of the DSM-5 criteria that can make up someone's BPD. Your symptoms might look different compared with another person's, and that's OK. But you're not alone in trying to manage these problems" (Project Air 2020).

Etiology: "It Is Not Your Fault, Nor Your Parents' Fault"

BPD results from an interaction between inherited temperamental and neurobiological dispositions in children and their caretaking environment. Its high heritability (~55%) means that families need to tailor their caregiving to adapt to the vulnerabilities of the patient's genetics (Distel et al. 2008; Gunderson et al. 2011b; Kendler et al. 2003; Torgersen et al. 2012). Neurologically, people with BPD tend to have an underactive prefrontal cortex, so they have fewer cognitive or thinking inhibitions, and a hyperreactive amygdala, so they are easily excited (Schulze et al. 2016). Effective therapies for BPD usually aim to promote activity in the prefrontal cortex to enhance thinking to evaluate perceptions and to manage the behaviors and feelings that are easily activated.

The increased sensitivity to stressors, especially those that are interpersonal, means that patients can get relief from structured and supportive environments. Parenting and peer behaviors have reciprocal effects on BPD symptom development in childhood and early adolescence. Harsh punishment and low warmth from parents can elicit BPD symptoms, such as fear of abandonment. In return, those same BPD symptoms may lead stressed parents to harsher punishments and difficulty expressing warmth, creating a self-perpetuating cycle. Similarly, bullying and rejection from peers predict BPD symptom severity, and more severe symptoms also predict bullying and rejection—another cycle (Stepp et al. 2014b; Winsper et al. 2017). To help young people with BPD manage their symptoms, validate their experiences while being clear about boundaries and expectations for change.

Course: "Change Takes Time, but Recovery Is Possible"

BPD traits rise during the early teenage years and decline linearly from mid-teens to late 20s (Johnson et al. 2000). During the adolescent phase, impulsivity, attention seeking, and dependency typically decrease, and social competence and self-control typically increase (Chanen and Thompson 2014). BPD symptoms can get better or worse depending on life situations (Conway et al. 2017), and for some teenagers, symptoms can fully resolve as they mature (Wright et al. 2016a). Most adult patients with BPD have symptom remission (about 28% after 2 years, 85% after 10 years) (Grilo et al. 2004; Gunderson et al. 2011a), and once remission is sustained, only about 15% relapse (Gunderson et al. 2011a; Zanarini et al. 2010). However, adults' symptom improvement is associated with only modest improvements in social functioning (only about one-third achieve full-time employment by 10 years) (Gunderson et al. 2011a).

Treatment: "You Have Options That Can Work"

Multiple early interventions have been shown to be effective at reducing self-harm, depression, and BPD symptoms in youths (Wong et al. 2020). Patients with BPD can improve with both specialized therapies such as dialectical behavior therapy for adolescents and mentalization-based treatment for adolescents, as well as less intensive treatments such as GPM for adolescents (GPM-A). For those who do not respond to GPM-A, more intensive BPD therapies can be an alternative. Because this treatment may be the patient and family's first encounter with mental health services, psychoeducation should include a discussion of the treatment's theory, duration, expectations, and confidentiality so the patient and family can anticipate the challenges ahead and remain engaged throughout (Desrosiers et al. 2020; see Chapter 4, "Getting Started").

Self-Care: "Your Job Is Growing Up, and Healthy Habits Can Help You Do That"

Adolescents' key developmental task is growing up to be their own unique person. This involves developing a sense of agency and independence. One way to promote autonomy is to discuss concrete ways in which adolescents can take care of themselves because a healthy lifestyle can both help adolescents become more self-sufficient and help them become more resilient in the face of difficult emotions and situations. Rather than being authoritarian, health professionals can make recommendations unapologetically with their rationale explained clearly, which the adolescent patient will need to consider, adapt, or reject. Key points that you can discuss are listed in Table 3–3. Clinicians should collaboratively discuss the pros and cons of different lifestyle choices, emphasizing that the adolescent's body and choices are their own, but sharing that "developing healthy habits will give you the best chance to accomplish your goals and live a life you want to live."

> To begin to feel better, it can be helpful to go back to basics. Our minds and bodies are connected, and our minds tend to feel better when our bodies are well rested, have necessary fuel, and are free of toxins. You are in charge of your body, and you can decide to make changes to strengthen yourself. Would you like to work together to try to get your sleep back on track?

Common Problems

Your Patient or the Parents Refuse the BPD Diagnosis

Patients might feel blamed for their problems, might feel attached to prior diagnoses from cherished treaters, or might perceive BPD pejoratively and therefore refuse to accept BPD as their diagnosis. If they are resistant, there is no need to push them: the priority is to agree on concrete treatment goals (e.g., "Let's try to change how you respond to stressful situations at school"). Collaborating on these issues successfully can help shift the focus of treatment to other, more BPD-specific problems such as rejection sensitivity, angry outbursts, and a sense of badness. Although these problems can be targeted without the patient's acceptance of the BPD diagnosis, it will still be useful to re-present the diagnosis again later on, for the reasons outlined above. The discussion of the diagnosis is important insofar as it helps patients understand themselves and guide treatment decisions. If the patient does not find the diagnosis relevant, ensuring that they understand the fundamental dynamics of BPD may still be a useful way to help the youth gain awareness and enhanced coping in the face of recurrent problems.

TABLE 3–3.   Areas for basic adolescent self-care

Lifestyle factor	Recommendations and fast facts
Sleep	Sleep 6–9 hours a night, around the same time every day
	• Sleep disturbance is associated with BPD and other psychiatric disorders in the teenage years (Brand and Kirov 2011; Wall et al. 2020).
	• Although sleep disturbances are normative in adolescence, teens with BPD have more variable sleep times and spend more time awake in bed than do teens without BPD (Huỳnh et al. 2016).
	• In one study, shorter sleep duration and later bedtime in early life were associated with BPD symptoms at ages 11–12 years (Morales-Muñoz et al. 2020).
Alcohol and drugs	Reduce or eliminate alcohol and drug use
	• Adolescents with BPD are four to nine times more likely than the general population to be dependent on alcohol, use tobacco daily, and use illicit substances (Scalzo et al. 2018).
	• Higher alcohol use is associated with more severe levels of BPD in adolescence (Lazarus et al. 2017).
	• BPD features predict later alcohol use problems (Stepp et al. 2005).
	• Increased BPD severity in adolescence contributes to earlier and quicker escalation of alcohol or drug use disorder symptoms, and problems with substance use can delay the normative decline in BPD symptoms (Bornovalova et al. 2018).
Nutrition	Maintain a balanced diet
	• A healthy diet can reduce stress and risk of depression in adolescents (Cairns et al. 2014; Cartwright et al. 2003).
Exercise	Exercise regularly
	• Physical activity contributes to positive cognitive and mental health outcomes in adolescents (Lubans et al. 2016).

TABLE 3–3.	Areas for basic adolescent self-care *(continued)*
Lifestyle factor	**Recommendations and fast facts**
Intimacy	Focus on school and friends over dating, and if dating, practice safe sex
	• Adolescents with BPD tend to engage in sexual relationships at a younger age, have a higher number of past-year sexual partners, have more casual relationships, practice unsafe sex during their first sexual experience, be coerced into unwanted sexual activity, be unclear about their sexual identity (Thompson et al. 2019a), and have increased relational insecurity (Lazarus et al. 2019).
	• Intense early exclusive romantic relationships predict heightened BPD symptoms (Lazarus et al. 2019).
	• Dating in middle and high school students is positively associated with alcohol, drug use, and self-harm. In one study, suicide attempts were positively associated with dating among seventh- and ninth-grade girls (Swahn et al. 2009).

Clinicians can present to families how the patient fits the criteria for BPD, while also being flexible in accommodating their perspective instead of insisting they accept the diagnosis:

> Your daughter has five of nine symptoms of BPD, so in the current moment she meets full criteria for the disorder. However, the development and consolidation of personality is in flux during adolescence, so it is hard to predict how things will progress. She may continue having BPD symptoms, she may develop other types of symptoms, or many of her problems may resolve with time. Whether we call it BPD or simply recognize that your daughter's core problem is maladaptive interpersonal and self function, we can see it as a chance for us to provide scaffolding for her personality to come together in a coherent way. Either way, we need to do the same thing: support her in managing her symptoms and getting a life outside treatment.

You Believe Your Patient Has BPD, but They Do Not Meet the DSM Threshold

Adolescents with both subthreshold (three symptoms) and full-syndrome (five symptoms) BPD show greater comorbidity and impairment in health-related quality of life; poorer social and occupational functioning; and more distress, risk-taking, self-injury, and suicidality compared with those without BPD (Kaess et al. 2017; Thompson et al. 2019b). Lowering the diagnostic cutoff for adolescents to three symptoms can help reach those who are at risk at an earlier stage before more intensive interventions are required because of severe life-interrupting and threatening episodes. According to the GPM model, the interpersonal BPD criteria (e.g., splits in self-image or in perceptions of others, fears of abandonment or aloneness, excessive rejection sensitivity) are most central and should be a focus of treatment even if adolescents do not meet full criteria for BPD. Often, these concerns are relevant to any adolescent with mental health vulnerabilities, with or without the diagnosis of BPD. When patients know that many others have this same set of problems, they can feel less alienated and alone.

Chapter 4

Getting Started

Teresa Carreño, M.D.
Gabrielle Ilagan, B.A.

Setting the Framework

When working with teens in good psychiatric management for adolescents (GPM-A), the clinician should conceptualize the patient as part of a family system, as in the following example from a meeting with the parents of a 12-year-old girl with borderline personality disorder (BPD):

> To start, I can meet with Amanda weekly and with you monthly to see if it helps. Let's not meet more frequently until we see if I can be useful to her and to you. We will know this by noticing if she feels better and if the tension at home improves. We will look for behavioral improvements in her anger and self-harm and see whether her relationships are getting better—slowly becoming more trusting and less controlling.

The structure of treatment usually involves weekly meetings with the teen and periodic meetings with parents. The structure is flexible on the basis of the patient's developmental age and the individual needs of the patient and family (Tables 4–1, 4–2, and 4–3). A core principle of GPM-A is that the frequency of sessions and duration of treatment are determined by whether the patient and family are finding the treatment useful and whether the patient is improving.

TABLE 4–1.   GPM-A framework

Sessions with the teen are held once weekly.

Parent work is a component (varies in form).

Duration depends on progress.

Adjunctive (split) treatments (family, medication, possibly group) are desirable.

Participation in school teams or clubs is encouraged.

Consultations and peer discussions are desirable.

Source.   Adapted from Gunderson JG, Links P: *Handbook of Good Psychiatric Management for Borderline Personality Disorder*, p. 28. Washington, DC, American Psychiatric Publishing, 2014. Copyright © 2014 American Psychiatric Publishing. Used with permission.

TABLE 4–2.   GPM-A framework and family involvement

Family involvement

Amount of involvement varies with the patient's developmental age.

Family members are collateral informants in the evaluative process.

Clinician provides diagnostic disclosure and psychoeducation.

Clinician provides referral to support systems (e.g., Family Connections network, NEABPD website).

When to meet with family

Evaluation

Diagnostic disclosure and psychoeducation

Setting the frame and frame adjustments

Discussion on limit setting

Troubleshooting

Times of important life decisions

Periodic treatment reviews (not only when problems arise)

Note.   NEABPD=National Education Alliance for Borderline Personality Disorder.

TABLE 4–3. **Treatment frame and family across adolescent development**

Ages 12–14 years

Parents are more involved.

Clinician discloses diagnosis to parents first.

Regular parent meetings should be held at least monthly and include psychoeducation about adolescent teen development and shifting parent roles.

Parent work may be primary and weekly in cases where the youth refuses treatment at the outset.

Intense acute presentations such as eating disorders and school refusal can be a presenting problem (Chanen et al. 2007; Chu et al. 2015)—then the primary focus of the family work is to get the teen to address the health crisis or to return to school.

Ages 15–17 years

Frequency of parent meetings should be monthly at the outset and may decrease as the patient and family improve.

Ages 18–21 years

Although legally adult, patients with BPD most often depend on family for emotional and financial support.

Family involvement with consent is most often a necessary part of the treatment frame:
• Evaluation
• Diagnostic disclosure and psychoeducation
• Setting the frame
• As needed

Ages 22–25 years

Family involvement with patient's consent as part of the frame is essential in patients who depend on family financially or emotionally.
Tailor family involvement to individual situation and need.

A common pattern to avoid is that of crises followed by increased care that feels reassuring in a manner that fosters more crises and a lack of improvement in the BPD symptoms over time. For example, after a careful assessment, in a meeting with 15-year-old Janet prior to a joint meeting with her parents to set the framework for a new treatment, you might say the following:

> Janet, this was your fifth visit to the emergency room this year. Although you feel better now, I am concerned that you have not made any progress in managing your intense reactions nor in attending school regularly. *I noticed something important in what you have been telling me.* You described that each time you have hurt yourself, it has been after someone you love has disappointed you [names examples]—*am I right? I had an idea about this and want to know what you think. I wonder if* when you feel disappointed in someone you love, you feel that no one cares and you quickly hurt yourself. Then, when someone shows they care by jumping to your rescue, *I can imagine* feeling a big relief and good that someone cares. *What do you think? [Listens openly and respectfully to her thoughts]* I want you to be OK. The problem is that you have not been learning other ways to help yourself feel better, so you are stuck in this cycle and this is not working. I will be meeting with you and your parents later today to try to figure out together what we might do differently to help you get unstuck.

Notice that Janet's pattern of maladaptive reactions to her interpersonal hypersensitivity is spelled out to her directly. She can consider it and decide whether or not it fits her experience. Importantly, Janet is being treated in a manner that respects her autonomy by making sure to acknowledge her feelings as her own, separate from the therapist's thoughts and feelings. The italics demonstrate how the clinician marks what Janet said as important, asking her opinion while listening openly and respectfully to her thoughts (see "Mentalization-Based Treatment for Adolescents" in Appendix A, "Relation of Good Psychiatric Management for Adolescents to Other Evidence-Based Treatments for Adolescent Borderline Personality Disorder").

If the patient does not agree with you, take no for an answer and work with what the patient tells you. Any approach that does not provide space for the teen's independent input is at risk of being superficially agreed to or rejected. In this example, the clinician meets with Janet first in order to begin to consolidate a working alliance with her as her own person. Janet now knows what will be discussed with her parents. Patient and family will be treated as accountable collaborators in a process of change.

Establish a collaborative relationship early on to build a working alliance with parents and youth. This alliance will serve as a stronghold that can anchor the therapy in difficult moments. Foster the development of this alliance at the outset and tend to it throughout the process of treatment. This can help prevent treatment dropout, a common problem in working with teens with BPD (Daly et al. 2010; Desrosiers et al. 2015; Gersh et al. 2017).

The presentation across this age group is variable, necessitating flexibility and creativity in structuring sessions. For example, if the youth is refusing to participate in therapy, work with parents can open an avenue for helpful intervention (see Case Vignette 1 in Chapter 9, "Case Illustrations"). Both patients and caregivers are helpful informants of progress. Their sense of how frequently it is helpful to meet can help guide the framework so long as the patient is improving. Meeting more than twice a week is not recommended. Review of the need for this level of frequency can be done by a consultant or in supervision. The increased level of emotional intensity created by meeting more frequently can become "too much" and increase dependency on treatment.

Constructive peer involvement in extracurricular activities such as school clubs or teams is recommended for teens as part of the frame of treatment. These social settings are developmentally important as places to practice relating with others and trying out new roles. They also provide material to discuss during sessions. Participation in extracurricular activities enhances a sense of peer belonging and better mental health in teens (Oberle et al. 2019; see Chapter 7, "Multimodal Treatments"). These activities are structured and have a common goal or interest and adult supervision. If this fails, then a second form of therapeutic involvement such as group therapy or self-help groups might be beneficial, although they may not be as beneficial in teens as in adults (Bo et al. 2020; see Chapter 7).

Communication between treaters is essential. The patient and family should be made aware that the treaters will need to communicate with each other as deemed necessary. Openness to the use of consultation is essential in treating teens with BPD. When the primary clinician is a psychiatrist, their role could include medication management, and the use of a consultant for complicated questions might also be helpful (see Chapter 6, "Pharmacotherapy and Comorbidity"). Another important aspect of GPM is case management by the primary clinician or collaboration with a case manager if needed. As the patient improves, increased engagement in school activities, teams, or clubs may necessitate flexibility in scheduling. Decreasing session frequency or using telehealth meetings can be considered. Constructive purposeful peer involvement is a significant sign of improvement and is a facilitator of healthy psychological development in teens.

Assessing Progress

Assessing progress and discussing whether change is occurring is an important role of the GPM-A clinician. Patients and parents are also encouraged to take an active role in monitoring change. Specific areas to monitor include improvement in subjective distress or dysphoria, behavior, interpersonal relationships, and social function (Table 4–4).

Notice your own feelings in the therapy:

- Am I understanding my patient and their parents better?
- Can I better predict how they are going to react? What makes them angry or what might trigger self-harm?
- Am I feeling more involved? Do I think about them between sessions; do I worry?
- Do the patient and family trust me more? Do they feel they can depend on me more?

If these changes are not happening, question the usefulness of the treatment.

If there is question as to the effectiveness of the treatment, do not hesitate to explicitly raise the question. Table 4–5 lists markers of change and offers guidelines as to when to question whether treatment is helping. There are many exceptions, however, and if treatment effectiveness is in question, consultation is recommended to consider the need to change treatment. This emphasizes the goal of treatment and the responsibility that all involved have to contribute to that outcome.

Parent Work and Building an Alliance

Essential elements of any therapy include the development of the patient's and family's trust that the therapist is well intentioned and their

TABLE 4-4. Expectable changes in teens

Target area	Changes	Relevant interventions
Subjective distress or dysphoria	↓ Anxiety and depression	Family work, support, situational changes ↑ Self-awareness
Behavior	↓ Self-harm, rages, promiscuity, suicidality, drug use	↑ Parental awareness of difficulties ↓ Parent negative emotion ↑ Awareness of self and interpersonal triggers ↑ Problem-solving strategies
Interpersonal relationships	↓ Devaluation ↑ Assertiveness ↑ Reciprocity ↓ Neediness ↑ Healthy dependency on therapist and others	↑ Mentalization ↑ Stability of attachment
Social function	School/work/home responsibilities and relationships	↓ Fear of failure and abandonment Coaching

Source. Adapted from Gunderson JG, Links P: *Handbook of Good Psychiatric Management for Borderline Personality Disorder.* Washington, DC, American Psychiatric Publishing, 2014, p. 29. Copyright © 2014 American Psychiatric Publishing. Used with permission.

inclination to follow the therapist's advice. The therapeutic alliance develops in the context of the therapist's careful and consistent listening and steadfast attempt to understand and validate the patient's and family's painful experiences. Table 4–6 describes the different levels and sequence of development of the therapeutic alliance.

When working with youths, it is essential to keep in mind that the youth is part of a larger family system and parents are critical to anchoring and maintaining any therapeutic process that takes place. Psychoeducation provides a shared construct through which the therapist, patient, and family can understand the teen's troubles, as discussed in Chapter 3, "Making the Diagnosis and Providing Psychoeducation."

TABLE 4–5.	When to question whether treatment is failing[a]

Time in treatment	Observation
Shorter term	
Weeks	Attendance is poor.
	Subjective distress is not better.
	You do not like the patient and/or caretakers.
Months	Patient or caretakers consistently disparage the therapy.
	Self-endangering events or activities of daily living (e.g., sleep, diet) worsen.
	Your empathy or understanding has not improved.
Longer term	
About 6 months	Level of self-endangering behaviors persists.
	Patient does not remember or use lessons from prior sessions.
	Patient has not increased engagement in school or work activities.
	Patient and parents do not recognize significance of adverse interpersonal events such as rejection or separations.

[a]Adapted from adult data.

Source.   Adapted from Gunderson JG, Links P: *Handbook of Good Psychiatric Management for Borderline Personality Disorder.* Washington, DC, American Psychiatric Publishing, 2014, p. 30. Copyright © 2014 American Psychiatric Publishing. Used with permission.

TABLE 4–6. Sequential forms of therapeutic alliance

Form of alliance	Description
Contractual (goals/roles)	Contractual alliance refers to setting the framework (schedule, fee, confidentiality) and establishing an agreement between patient and therapist on treatment goals and their roles in achieving them (see section "Setting the Framework" in this chapter). This form is relevant to all modalities and can be established in the first session, but it may take two or three sessions.
Relational (affective/ empathic)	Relational alliance refers to a therapist's perception of the patient as likable and understandable and to the patient's experience of the therapist as caring, understanding, genuine, and likable. This form of alliance can develop very quickly and should have developed by 6 months. If sustained, it is a corrective experience.
Working (cognitive/ motivational)	In a working alliance, the patient is a reliable collaborator who can recognize unwanted pain-inducing observations by a therapist as being well intended. This form of alliance grows gradually, is especially relevant to individual psychotherapies, and varies within sessions.

Source. Adapted from Gunderson JG, Links P: *Handbook of Good Psychiatric Management for Borderline Personality Disorder.* Washington, DC, American Psychiatric Publishing, 2014, p. 32. Copyright © 2014 American Psychiatric Publishing. Used with permission.

Parent work is an essential part of the treatment plan when working with teens. After psychoeducation, the next basic step will be to socialize the patient and family to the process of therapy in order to establish what is to be expected and the nature of a therapeutic relationship. As part of this process, predict a possible treatment rupture. This could serve to inoculate the treatment from early treatment dropout (de Haan et al. 2014; Desrosiers et al. 2015; Kazdin 1996; Midgley et al. 2016).

Jody, you and I and your parents will work together as we agreed. In our meetings, you and I will try to really understand you and find ways that are helpful to meeting the goals we agreed on. I will also work with you and your parents to try to help you understand each other better so that they can be more helpful to you. Within reason, what you and I discuss will be private. I will share with your parents what we are working on, what is expected, how the therapy should be set up, any issues dealing with safety, and other things that you and I agree would be helpful for them to know.

I will try hard to be useful and helpful to you and your family. There may come a time that something happens between us that you don't agree with. If that happens, it will be very important for you to try to tell me. Do you think you would be able to do that? I really care about that and would want to know so that we can try to figure it out together.

As illustrated in the dialogue above, disclosure of information is addressed with patients and parents at the beginning of treatment. By and large, parents will be told when there is a threat to safety or to life, even if the teen disagrees with the disclosure. They also will be informed of the structure and expectations of treatment. They will not be informed about what happens in every session. When pertinent, develop a safety plan at the beginning of treatment in collaboration with the patient and parents (see Chapter 5, "Managing Suicidality and Nonsuicidal Self-Injury"). Acknowledge and address the chief complaints of both the patient and the parents. Parents are also a valuable source of collateral information about progress in treatment. It is important to be aware that parents and families often suffer a high level of subjective distress or trauma, and their needs must be identified and addressed (Bailey and Grenyer 2014; Hoffman et al. 1999; Lawn and McMahon 2015). Emphasize good self-care for the carers as an essential part of the treatment of BPD.

> Taking care of your teen's challenges can sometimes wear you down. This is why it is important for you to be attuned to your own reserves, much like how on a plane, we are told to put on our oxygen masks first and then to help others.

Initially, parent meetings can be scheduled predictably about once a month for treatment reviews, not only when problems arise. At first, focus on psychoeducation, coaching the family on decreasing the intensity of expressed emotion, improving awareness of stress vulnerability in the youth, and decreasing stress by making stepwise goals. Guidance is given to make sure the parents and the teen spend time together that is not focused on problems. Make sure families know not to forgo good times for the family and connecting with others. These family interventions have the intent of increasing parent warmth and decreasing negativity (Stepp et al. 2014b), which can improve BPD symptoms in the teen. The frequency of meetings can be adjusted over time depending on each family's needs.

> Your teen is particularly sensitive to stress, especially in close relationships, so it can be helpful to keep the "emotional thermometer" at home on the cooler side. This will help him keep his thinking more in line. It is important not to expect too much of him early on and to gradually reset goals when he is ready, as gains are made. In the midst of all this, remember to plan for good times and don't shy away from friends and family.

Teens and parents are navigating a developmental period when the teen's need of their parents is in flux. Although teens depend on their parents, they often feel uncomfortable about needing or accepting their help. This is a time when treatment may be refused by the teen, particularly if it is seen as an extension of parental influence. As the youth enters mid to later adolescence, more responsibility shifts to the teen. At every age, the youth needs to be approached as an individual with agency, and their feelings and thoughts should be acknowledged as valid by the therapist and family.

Teens and their parents will often have different treatment goals. Ask the teen what they think about the parents' goals. Take the teen's goals seriously and find points of overlap between the goals of parents and youth. This common ground can serve as a springboard for both parents and teens to begin to collaborate with each other and with the clinician in the treatment process. However, agreement with the teen's ideas or actions is not always expected nor desirable. Walk the fine line of validating while being free to disagree (Garland et al. 2004). (For a more specific approach, see Appendix D, "Guidelines for Families.") The interventions in the following subsections also foster the development of the therapeutic alliance and the patient's collaborative spirit to work with the therapist toward improvement.

Session Content and Relational Hypersensitivity

Because of their intense temperament and interpersonal hypersensitivity, as well as the naturally intensified relational environment of adolescence, teens with BPD are in a chronic state of emotional overstimulation, and they relate to others erratically and often negatively (Jovev et al. 2012; von Ceumern-Lindenstjerna et al. 2010). They are at greater risk of being bullied (Jopling et al. 2016) and feeling misunderstood. Their experience of themselves in relationships can be negative and confusing. GPM-A sessions focus on increasing awareness of patients' relational hypersensitivity in their interactions with peers, family, and the therapist and how their reaction to others influences how they are perceived and treated.[1] As relational awareness of self and other improves, teens' manner of relating to others becomes more coherent. The increasingly consistent and positive experience with others fosters a more coherent experience of themselves and facilitates their development of a sense of self, a critical developmental task of adolescence.

John, when David looked upset, you thought he was mad at you and you felt hurt, so you blocked him. Then he told your friends and they blew you off and you felt horribly. Later, it turned out he was upset because he lost a game. This is a good example of overreading and then reacting. When you blocked him, he probably felt hurt and confused and reached out to friends who didn't understand why you would have blocked him. Then they got cold and you felt worse and misunderstood. The next time someone looks upset, how might you handle it differently, knowing you have a tendency to overread?

Homework

It is important to encourage teens to actively focus on the issues you discuss in their life between sessions. It can be helpful to mention having thought about them and to make reference to a previous session when something related surfaces, creating continuity between sessions and encouraging patients to feel their presence in your mind and to increase your presence in theirs. Homework is recommended to help structure the therapy focus outside the meeting.

I'd like you to be able to make sense of yourself and your life. Have you noticed a pattern that seems to recur whenever you start school? Whenever I go away? Or at other times?

How does this relate to our last session? To peer situations? To your past experiences?

---

[1]One vulnerability found particularly in teens with BPD is the tendency to *overread* relational cues—they "make assumptions about other people's mental states that go so far beyond observable data that the average observer will struggle to see how they are justified" (Sharp et al. 2013, p. 4), which is also known as *hypermentalizing*. This can lead to intense negative emotional reactions and impulsive behaviors that can trigger social rejection.

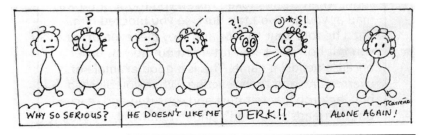

FIGURE 4–1.   Interpersonal hypersensitivity cartoon.

Therapy Journal or Folder

Therapy sessions can be emotionally intense. You may suggest a journal from the outset that can be decorated meaningfully by the teen. Homework can be written here together with diagrams and take-aways during sessions. This can help the teen hold on to the homework and content of the session better.

Autobiography and Creative Expression

Adolescence is a developmental time of increased creativity, and this can be used in treatment homework (Shaw 1981). For example, some teens enjoy drawing or writing poetry. This can be a way to express life stories or to organize relational experiences between sessions that can later be discussed in session. An autobiography can also be a useful way to organize past experiences and build a narrative. You may begin by asking the patient to draw a family tree around which a life story can be elaborated over time.

Relational Patterns

Get creative in exploring relationship patterns. For example, when a misunderstanding has happened in a relationship and there has been repair, develop (perhaps sketch) a template with the patient that demonstrates how relational hypersensitivity led to an intense emotional reaction and a reactive interpersonal response that caused increased misunderstanding and sense of distance. With adolescents, it can be most helpful to focus on what helped to repair the situation, looking out for moments when the teen showed strength and prosocial behavior. For example, in collaboration with the teen, you might draw a cartoon such as the one illustrated in Figure 4–1, then draw a second cartoon with the last three frames empty. Together with the patient, figure out how to use what they learned from the repair to make the outcome different next time. This can be

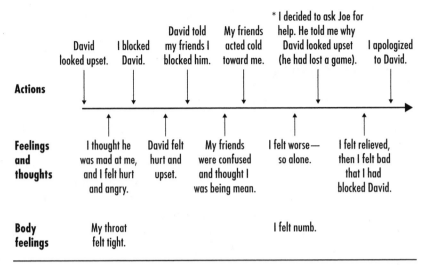

FIGURE 4–2. **Interpersonal chain analysis.**

This example is from a dialogue bubble in earlier subsection "Session Content and Relational Hypersensitivity." The asterisk indicates a moment of strength and prosocial behavior.

helpful later when ruptures occur in treatment. Repair of unintended ruptures in the relationship with the therapist can lead to progress in BPD treatment (Daly et al. 2010; Gersh et al. 2017).

Detailing a Recent Crisis

Develop a chain analysis to help the teen think about a recent crisis and be curious about the triggering event and the sequence of thoughts, feelings, and reactions that led to the crisis. The idea is to identify in increasing detail points in the sequence that could be used to interrupt this chain of events the next time there is a triggering circumstance in order to avert a crisis. In Figure 4-2, notice the moment of strength and prosocial behavior that is highlighted. Focusing on these healthy moments of resilience in the therapy session and helping the teen to reproduce them on purpose is a particularly effective way to help teens change maladaptive patterns of relating.

Structured Forms

Any type of self-assessment that better elaborates and characterizes the patient's experience can be used, such as personality questionnaires, mood monitors, and computerized research instruments. Useful homework includes filling out safety plans (see Chapter 5, Figure 5–3) or monitoring how symptoms respond to interventions or medications. Apps may be used to journal, rate, or help the teen cope with experiences in vivo between sessions.

Setting Goals

The Goal of Setting a Goal

Teens with BPD in crisis may be unable to meaningfully set goals at the outset of treatment because of a profound distrust or inability to read their own feelings accurately. For them, a goal of therapy is to become able to establish goals to promote self-direction. Initially, goals should be short term and attainable, such as leaving a stressful situation or calling for support, improving sleep, or trying to go back to school. Break down goals so that the first step becomes manageable. Each step can improve the teen's sense of mastery and reinforce efforts to change.

Getting Back on Track Toward Developing "a Life Worth Living"

An overarching treatment goal is to help the adolescent get back on track developmentally. Teens are developing their capacities to work, play, and love, so it is important to minimize obstructions to normal development that can be a consequence of the emotional, behavioral, and relational symptoms of BPD. Outcomes that matter include increasing capacity for learning, relatedness, and trust. These gains are believed to facilitate development of self-identity (Fonagy et al. 2019). To monitor progress, assess the teen's ability to attend and perform adequately in school, manage relationships with peers, and discover interests and talents. Attempt to increase resilience by helping teens understand their relational hypersensitivity and the effect of their reactiveness on peers and parents. This motivates the development of more adaptive ways to identify and address relational triggers with the intent to set up a positive feedback loop helping to transform a vicious cycle of relatedness into a virtuous one.

Other Interventions

Other techniques to use in working with teens with BPD include the following.

- Include the teen in planning appointments, even if parents keep the teen's schedule. If resistant, the teen might initially agree to a limited number of appointments, perhaps six, at which time the need for further appointments can be revisited. These appointments can be included in the therapy notebook and be crossed off. By the last scheduled session, evaluate together whether the meetings are helping to help inform the teen how to proceed with treatment.

- Call about missed appointments, particularly early in treatment. Missing appointments is expected and not necessarily an indication of treatment refusal (Chanen et al. 2014). Early parent work can focus on facilitating therapy attendance by addressing impediments to meeting regularly.
- Advise "growing many roots" (Figure 4–3). Teens with BPD may be strongly drawn to romantic relationships, but early romantic relationships may confer risk to these teens, perhaps by evoking too much emotional stimulation (Lazarus et al. 2019). This risk may be offset by having other interests, too.

> I hear you when you tell me your relationship with Izzy is your happiness, and I am glad you are happy. However, I am reminded that people are a lot like trees: Our roots are the things that matter to us. A tree is much stronger when it has many roots, so if one gets loose, the others still hold it steady. Roots can be school, hobbies, friends, family, and in your case, Izzy, too.

- Talk about "growing up." For example: "You are busy growing up and becoming an adult. It is a privilege to be beside you in this process. I'm on your side as you go through this process of growing up, which ends only when you are 25." This gives teens a sense of participation in the business of growing up so that they want to do their part in maturing.
- Focus on patterns of relatedness that might increase the probability of social rejection (Dixon-Gordon et al. 2011; Sharp and Fonagy 2015). Social rejection is a significant factor that merits clinical attention (Sharp

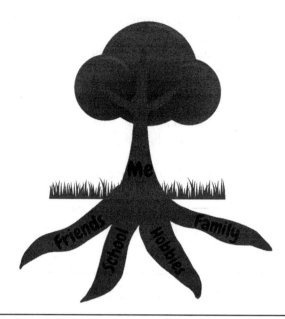

FIGURE 4–3.   Growing roots.

and Fonagy 2015; Wolke et al. 2012). Often, teens with BPD are not aware that their hyperreactivity toward others when feeling rejected can cause people to react angrily or to withdraw. Overreading, for example, is an important focus of clinical attention in and between sessions (see dialogue bubble in section "Homework"). Consider suggesting that the teen check with others about whether their interpretation of a situation seems like "too much."

- Case management as needed, such as helping an embarrassed teen compose a text to a tutor after having missed a session or arranging support for return to school after a crisis, is often helpful. This must be done with discretion and only with appropriate consent if feasible. Larger considerations might include advocating for neuropsychological testing for a teen who displays executive functioning deficits; addressing the need for accommodations at school, for tutoring, or for alternative school placement when appropriate; or identifying medical needs.
- Attend to family needs: referrals to Family Connections, a social support and education network for families (see "National Education Alliance for Borderline Personality Disorder (NEABPD)" in Appendix E, "Online Resources") or multifamily groups where available and indi-

vidual or family therapy referrals or social work referrals when social needs are identified.

- Facilitate necessary but difficult family communications on limit setting, troubleshooting, times of transition, or important life decisions.
- Attend to any identified medical needs, including eating and sleep hygiene (see Chapter 3, Table 3–3).
- Address and actively treat comorbidities, particularly ADHD (Biskin 2013; Golubchik et al. 2008) (see Chapter 6).

Intersession Availability

> If you have an emergency, I want to be available to you, and I want you to grow trust that I care that you will be OK. Because it's not possible for me to always be available, we should talk about other options, too. What other options can we think of?

Your patient and family or caretakers have managed and can most likely continue to manage personal crises between scheduled sessions (Gunderson 1996; Nadort et al. 2009). The issue of intersession availability should be addressed when the family clearly cannot manage or when you are asked by the patient or family. The caretakers and patients should remain as responsible for the patient's well-being as possible.

Figure 4–4 outlines a strategy for managing availability between sessions. Special clinical attention is needed if the teen and family did not call when help was needed or if the teen or family called about something that could have waited until the next session. If no call was made during an emergency, this opens an opportunity to explore with the teen and family the impediments to getting help. If a call was made for something that did not seem to be a crisis, the next session can be used to explore the patient's fear of aloneness, lack of caring, or excessive use of others to self-soothe. After you, the patient, and the family together have come to a better understanding of what happened, a plan can be crafted collaboratively with the patient or family for the next time a similar situation arises.

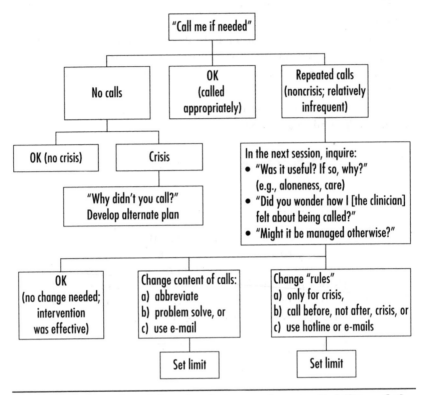

FIGURE 4–4. **Algorithm for intersession availability of the therapist.**

Source.   Adapted from Gunderson JG, Links P: *Handbook of Good Psychiatric Management for Borderline Personality Disorder*, p. 31. Washington, DC, American Psychiatric Publishing, 2014. Copyright © 2014 American Psychiatric Publishing. Used with permission.

Uncommonly, a situation may arise in which a limit needs to be set.

> Please understand that I cannot humanly be available to my patients on an unlimited basis, and responding to your calls has become too hard for me. Let's think together about other ways that you can get help.

Technology has opened avenues for communication. Electronic messages with patients and families can be used judiciously for communications about appointment changes or logistics to convey homework and not-too-private messages. Electronic communication can provide a calming sense of continuity of relational connectedness over time, which is often a challenge for patients with BPD. It is helpful to set up an understanding that nonadministrative messages will be discussed at the next meeting and not responded to immediately. This being said, privacy is less secure online, and urgent or very private communications should be discouraged. These discussions provide a good opportunity to help teens think about the limitations of electronic communication and remember to practice and generalize wiser use of e-messaging.

It is not sustainable to expect 24/7 availability for recurrent emergencies. Relational contact has a soothing effect for patients with BPD and must be used judiciously. Excessive need for soothing contact is often problematic to patients in their relationships with others, where they may be perceived as "too needy." Help patients develop a framework to self-soothe and cope with urges to self-harm (see the discussion of safety planning in Chapter 5) that does not revolve around reassuring contact with others. Encouraging contact by inviting calls without crises or providing excessive supportive listening can be counterproductive. Intersession contact should be addressed in the following session, and its necessity, value, and possible alternatives can then be discussed. Educating parents about this issue can also be helpful. Any patient or family who insists on 24/7 contact should be referred to a treatment team or higher level of care that has the capacity to manage this level of need.

Common Problems

Changing Therapists

Problems may arise when you are in a role to evaluate a patient already in therapy and conclude that the existing therapy is either ineffective or harmful, but the patient or treater do not agree. The therapist might take it personally as a criticism of their competence or character. In these situations, it is helpful to depersonalize the criticism and point out the lack of improvement in subjective distress, self-harm, or suicidality or the use of emergency and inpatient services. Treatment failures can happen, even in the hands of experienced and skilled clinicians. If the patient or family alone is resisting the change, it may be to avoid a painful separation. When this is the case, a follow-up meeting in perhaps 1 or 2 months with the previous treater may be helpful. Another idea is to resume the treatment when specified changes have occurred, for example, when the patient stops cutting or resumes attending school. It is often enough if the previous therapist supports the change or is encouraged to place limits on their ongoing availability. If both patient and treater do not agree with the change, then there may be no alternative other than to document your opinion and obtain consultation or ongoing supervision.

Patient or Family Refuses to Accept the Framework

Initially, the framework should be flexible. Although certain issues can impede the success of treatment, they may change as a therapeutic alliance develops. Examples of such issues include withholding legal consent for you to speak with prior treaters or family members (late teens) or refusal to commit to meeting weekly, to address any goals, to seek help when suicidal, or to stop alcohol or drug use. Only when these issues impair your ability to be helpful should you end the treatment. Some refusals are not workable; these include persistent intoxication, nonattendance, nonpayment, or refusal to adopt a safety plan when a patient is in serious danger (see section "Common Problems" in Chapter 5).

You Don't Like Your Patient or the Family

Patients with BPD may present with preconceived negative notions of clinicians, and they often view and speak about their parents in a negative light. In this context, negative feelings can be triggered in the clinician toward patients and/or their family. It is helpful to suspend judgment and try to understand the patient and family member from the context of their own perspective. If the clinician's negative feelings persist after a few sessions, it may be difficult to back out, particularly if the patient and family do not desire to change treaters. If the reason for your dislike is universal and would interfere with treatment, it should be discussed. Examples of such reasons include patient hygiene, silence, or disrespect or dismissiveness on the part of the patient or family. If your feelings are more of a personal nature (countertransference), consultation with a colleague or therapist is recommended. Examples of such issues include appearance, politics, dependency, or hostility on the part of the patient. If, after consultation, you feel that your aversion remains an impediment to treatment, you may inform the patient or family that you consider yourself a bad match because of your limitations and that they deserve to work with someone who will be better able to help them.

> Mr. and Mrs. Smith, I have thought very carefully about your needs and my ability to meet them and have come to the realization that I am not a good match to help you and Jeremy. I am really sorry. At the same time, I realize that you deserve a therapist who is able to meet your needs. For this reason, I feel it is in your best interest that you find a better match. If I can be of help facilitating this, I will certainly try.

You Will Be Unavailable for an Extended Time

The same principles apply as described earlier (see section "Intersession Availability"). As much as possible, the family and patient are considered capable of planning and being responsible for any treatment contacts that may be needed in your absence. Coverage should be arranged if you feel it is clinically warranted or if the patient or family wants it. You may make yourself available by phone or e-mail if it does not interfere with your plans. However, the oxygen mask metaphor applies to clinicians too. Pay clinical attention to the period of time preceding and following your absence. Adolescents with BPD are sensitive to relational disconnects, and although unintended, your absence tends to trigger negative feelings and reactions to the feelings.

Chapter 5

Managing Suicidality and Nonsuicidal Self-Injury

Marcos Croci, M.D.

Eduardo Martinho Jr., M.D., Ph.D.

Marcelo Brañas, M.D.

SELF-HARM AND SUICIDALITY are hallmark symptoms of borderline personality disorder (BPD) in both adolescents and adults (Table 5–1), bringing attention to the possibility of a BPD diagnosis. Although self-harm, or nonsuicidal self-injury (NSSI), is not unique to BPD (Table 5–2), its presence in adolescence may be an early sign of the disorder, especially if it is recurrent (Ghinea et al. 2019).

The average age of onset of NSSI for individuals with BPD is 13 years, significantly earlier than in those without the diagnosis (Groschwitz et al. 2015). One in three adults with BPD report first self-injuring before age 13 (Zanarini et al. 2006). Patients engage in NSSI to decrease negative emotions, to handle dissociative experiences, or to punish themselves (Sadeh et al. 2014). There is no intention to die. However, the presence of NSSI significantly increases the risk of suicide attempts (Scott et al. 2015). Self-injury may be associated with abnormalities in the areas of the brain implicated in pain processing, which in turn may diminish fear of more severe self-injury through habituation (Reitz et al. 2015; Schmahl et al. 2006). Over time, this pattern lowers the inhibitions against suicide attempts (Hamza et al. 2012; Nock et al. 2006).

Suicidality (i.e., suicidal thoughts, behavior), on the other hand, is characterized by the motivation to end one's life, even if ambivalent. BPD has long been associated with a significant percentage of completed suicides in adolescents (Rich and Runeson 1992; Runeson and Beskow 1991), contradicting the belief that attempted suicides by individuals with BPD are less severe. Although this behavior requires ongoing clinical attention, self-injurious and suicidal behaviors are expected to improve early in the treatment.

A major responsibility clinicians bear in their work with adolescents with BPD is the management of safety concerns. A number of intensive evidence-based treatments for adults with BPD effectively address suicidality and self-harm. Most clinicians working with adolescents will not have such specialized training. Good psychiatric management (GPM) encourages clinicians to rely on what they probably already know about the management of safety, integrated with an understanding of the interpersonal hypersensitivity model to assess level of risk and indicated level of care. Working with self-harming and suicidal patients can be a source of worry and liability. Factors that increase and decrease risk for liability can be managed effectively and responsibly by following standards of care and seeking consultation from colleagues (Table 5–3). When utilizing standards of care and current scientific findings about suicide and self-harm in adolescents with BPD, health professionals can demonstrate a clear foundation for responsible clinical reasoning.

Impending Self-Endangering Behaviors

As noted in Chapter 2, "Overall Principles," GPM's model of interpersonal hypersensitivity explains a pathway of events that lead to both self-harming

---

TABLE 5–1. **Borderline personality disorder's "behavioral specialty": suicidality and self-harm**

Suicide is the second-leading cause of death in adolescents and young adults (ages 10–24 years) in the United States (Heron 2019).

• Studies have shown that about 10%–40% of youths (ages 13–29 years) who completed suicide had BPD (Marttunen et al. 1991; Rich and Runeson 1992).

Follow-back studies have found a rate of 3%–10% of completed suicide among adults with BPD (Paris and Zweig-Frank 2001). However, a large prospective study has shown a rate of 6% over 24 years of follow-up (Temes et al. 2019).

• Individuals of younger age, from adolescence to third decade, appear to be at higher risk (Pompili et al. 2005).

About 75%–95% of adolescents with BPD engage in NSSI (Andrewes et al. 2019; Goodman et al. 2017).

• Self-harm is often a soothing method, but it is associated with increased risk of suicidality.

• NSSI includes cutting, punching, burning, and banging heads.

Suicide attempts are frequent, with rates up to 75% in the adolescent BPD population (Goodman et al. 2017).

• BPD uniquely predicts suicide attempts in adolescents (Scott et al. 2015).

Suicidal acts are usually ambivalent.

• Interpersonal connection decreases the risk: "If rescued, I want to live. If not, I prefer to die."

Impulsivity also plays a role in adolescent suicidality (Yen et al. 2013).

• These patients act while experiencing strong emotions (Fossati 2015; Kaess et al. 2014).

Comorbid major depression and substance abuse increase suicide risk (Kolla et al. 2008).

Interpersonal stressors trigger self-harm and suicidality in adolescents with BPD (Andrewes et al. 2019).

Note. BPD=borderline personality disorder; NSSI=nonsuicidal self-injury.

Source. Adapted from Gunderson and Links 2014, p. 38.

TABLE 5–2.   **Overview of nonsuicidal self-injury in non-BPD population**

Nonsuicidal self-injury (NSSI) is the direct and deliberate self-inflicted damage of body tissue without suicidal intention or socially sanctioned purpose (Brown and Plener 2017). This definition excludes other self-destructive behaviors such as substance abuse or eating disorders and culturally accepted self-injury, such as body piercing and tattoos (Lloyd-Richardson et al. 2007). Deliberate self-harm is another term seen in the literature that encompasses self-injury or self-poisoning regardless of suicidal intent (Carter et al. 2016).

NSSI is common in youths. Its prevalence in adolescence (ages 10–17) and young adulthood (ages 18–24) is 17% and 13%, respectively (Swannell et al. 2014). Studies have shown an increase in NSSI prevalence during young adolescence, with a decrease in late adolescence throughout young adulthood (Plener et al. 2015). Most adolescents' self-injury resolves spontaneously; however, some youths, especially those experiencing mental health problems, may continue this behavior until adulthood (Moran et al. 2012).

NSSI is associated with several mental disorders, other than BPD, such as anxiety disorders, depression, substance use disorders, eating disorders, PTSD, conduct disorders, oppositional defiant disorder, and other personality disorders; however, it may also be present in individuals without these comorbidities (Glenn and Klonsky 2013; Nock and Prinstein 2005). This finding resulted in the proposal of a separate nosological category, nonsuicidal self-injury, in section III of the *Diagnostic and Statistical Manual of Mental Disorders*, 5th Edition (DSM-5; American Psychiatric Association 2013), as a condition for further study (for an overview, see Zetterqvist 2015).

The first step in providing care for patients with NSSI is assessment (Plener et al. 2016), which includes physical examination (e.g., signs of infection, tetanus vaccine status, necessity of somatic treatment) and collection of history (e.g., origin, method, severity, and frequency of NSSI; psychiatric comorbidity; special attention to suicidality). The clinician's stance is also critical when facing adolescents who self-injure; the clinician should respond with supportive concern but should not overreact. A recommendation for caregivers is responding with concern and interest, being careful to not be dismissive but also trying not to be so focused on the behavior alone (or controlling it) out of context with the stressful experiences and emotions that preceded it. This approach is valid for patients with or without BPD. Contextualizing these behaviors in terms of patients' broader life difficulties, addressing precipitants, and considering environmental influences (e.g., family, colleagues, school, social media) are also important.

TABLE 5–2. **Overview of nonsuicidal self-injury in non-BPD population *(continued)***

The first line of treatment for NSSI is outpatient psychotherapy (Ougrin et al. 2015). Patients presenting solely with NSSI will rarely need hospitalization, and medications alone will not address self-injury. Evidence-based interventions include dialectical behavior therapy for adolescents, mentalization-based treatment for adolescents, and cognitive-behavioral therapy; however, these options often are unaccessible. Nevertheless, common factors across treatment approaches provide guidance. These include building commitment and motivation for treatment, providing psychoeducation for the patient and family about NSSI (e.g., what does it mean, how to react), increasing parental support and effective monitoring, identifying factors that trigger or maintain the behavior, treating comorbidities, and providing behavioral coping skills and problem-solving as alternatives to self-injuring (Carter et al. 2016; Plener et al. 2016).

Note.   BPD=borderline personality disorder.

TABLE 5–3. **Liability concerns in treating self-endangering behaviors in patients with borderline personality disorder**

The risk of liability is low (<1%) and diminishes among experienced therapists.

There is an increased risk of liability with poor management of the clinician-patient relationship. Careful attention should be paid to countertransference enactments such as unrealistic availability, punitive hostility, personal involvement, and illusions of omniscience or omnipotence.

Liability can be minimized by

• Careful documentation, mainly risk assessments and clinical decisions (Packman et al. 2004; Paris 2004)

• Discussing and consulting with colleagues or split treatments (Gunderson and Links 2014)

• Involving the family in psychoeducation (e.g., how suicidality occurs, suicide rates) and suicidal management (e.g., warning signs) (Gutheil 2004)

• Establishing a healthy relationship with the family (Packman et al. 2004)

• Showing support for the family after suicidal behavior (Gutheil 2004)

Source.   Adapted from Gunderson and Links 2014, p. 39.

states and more concerning suicidal states. Although threats to connectedness to others will elicit self-harming states, contact, however conflictual or aggravated, may relieve the patient with BPD from feeling abandoned. In contrast, when others withdraw from the patient completely and the patient is alone and truly despairing, then more concerning suicidality can arise. When others intervene, this can reconstitute the patient with BPD to a more connected and workable state. Often this kind of intervention takes the form of hospitalization, which, although containing, does not serve as an effective treatment plan over time. Hospitalization presents a unilateral solution to the patient's problems in a way that does not empower patients to participate in the management of their own safety. GPM's interpersonal hypersensitivity model guides clinicians to involve patients in their own rescue. (See section "Involving Patients in Their Safety With Psychoeducation, Safety Planning, and Coping Skills.")

The central principle for managing safety is to respond with concerned attention. Do not avoid the issue. Refrain from using a judgmental stance. This opens the path for empathy and exploration, helping the patient to vent and feel less lonely (Gunderson 2008). This alone can be an effective intervention in itself and can help decrease risk.

Assessing Suicidality and Dangerousness

In addition to providing emotional support, the clinician's primary task is to assess the dangerousness of the situation. The acute-on-chronic model (Figure 5–1) helps clinicians evaluate acute factors of immediate risk, layered on preexisting factors to guide their decisions about chronically impulsive and suicidal patients (Links et al. 2003).

Differentiating suicidality from self-harm is the most crucial step in evaluating safety. If the behavior is interpreted as truly dangerous instead of as deliberate self-soothing or a cry for help, clinicians are prone to perform excessive suicide assessments, reinforcing the nonadaptive use of suicidal threats. This pattern can cause you to hospitalize unnecessarily. However, if you respond with hostility or indifference, the risk of suicidality can escalate. Although NSSI is not suicidal, you can pay attention to sudden changes in its pattern and increases in its severity because these can signal an increase in risk (Andrewes et al. 2018).

The context in which these behaviors occur is often interpersonal (see Figure 2–1 in Chapter 2, "Overall Principles"). The patient may be in a clear crisis with suicidal ideation and a plan or may be desperately impulsive

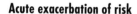

Acute exacerbation of risk

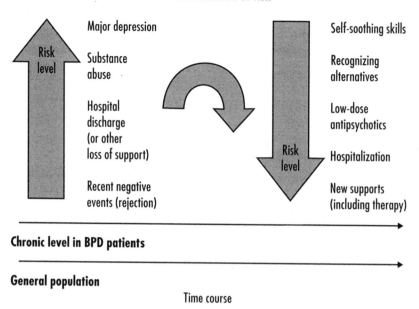

FIGURE 5–1. **Acute-on-chronic suicide risk.**

In patients with borderline personality disorder (BPD), the acute-on-chronic level of suicide risk (curved arrow) can change more quickly than it does in the general population and can be modified by several factors that can cause (upward arrow) and several that might reduce (downward arrow) an acute exacerbation of risk. *Source.* Reprinted from Gunderson JG, Links P: *Handbook of Good Psychiatric Management for Borderline Personality Disorder.* Washington, DC, American Psychiatric Publishing, 2014, p. 40. Copyright © 2014 American Psychiatric Publishing. Used with permission.

and affectively unstable with no explicit intention to die. In all of these situations, you can get the facts and understand the impending crisis (see interpersonal chain analysis in subsection "Nonsuicidal Self-Injury or Nonfatal Suicide Attempts" and example in Chapter 4, "Getting Started"). Environmental stressors should be examined, such as family conflict, peer isolation, bullying, or even negative experiences on social media (Links et al. 2003; Marchant et al. 2017).

Clinicians should assess and target sleep problems associated with suicidal behaviors in adolescents (Mars et al. 2019). Although comorbidity (e.g., major depression) may be a contributing factor, adolescents with BPD have trouble sleeping independent of other disorders. Insomnia can increase affective instability and impulsivity, thus increasing vulnerability to the interpersonal cascade toward suicidality (Huỳnh et al. 2016; Winsper and Tang 2014).

Patients with BPD have difficulty identifying emotions and communicating distress, especially in their adolescent years. Often, they may say that they want to disappear or that they are suicidal, and the clinician is left questioning whether the patient has a real intent to act on these thoughts. One strategy is to develop a personal method of rating the patient's level of emotional distress or suicidal risk. For example, a *feeling thermometer* graphic can be provided to help the teen evaluate their level of distress on a scale from 0 (a state of calm) to 10 (the highest emotional pain ever felt; Spirito et al. 2011). Then, the clinician and patient can figure out at which level of distress the teen loses self-control. This tool teaches self-awareness and self-control by using a continuous distress level instead of "all-or-nothing" thinking. It helps patients stop and think about emotions and teaches them to communicate better with their support network and therapist. Additionally, it can help tailor coping skills (e.g., taking deep breaths when feelings are getting out of hand, self-soothing before the distress goes even higher).

Safety contracts are not empirically supported and can give a false sense of safety for clinicians. A contract cannot replace risk assessment and can undermine trust because it may indicate therapist insecurity and concern for liability. Dialectical behavior therapy asks patients to leave suicide "off the table," which may help generate commitment to work collaboratively on alternatives but offers no guarantees (even for liability).

Selecting the Appropriate Level of Care

An algorithm for selecting the appropriate level of care is depicted in Figure 5–2. Outpatient care is preferred because it provides the opportunity to address recurrent suicidal or self-harming problems in the context of the patient's daily life rather than in the context of a highly supervised treatment setting. In the absence of intermediate levels of care (e.g., residential, partial hospital), short-term hospitalization should be considered when self-endangering behaviors are judged to be dangerous. The main principle in deciding whether or not to hospitalize is to weigh potential benefits (e.g., safety) and harms (e.g., regression, secondary gain) (Vijay and Links 2007).

If hospitalization occurs, it is essential to keep the focus on what prompted the self-destructive process, assuming interpersonal stressors may play a key role. It is also an opportunity to increase patient-family under-

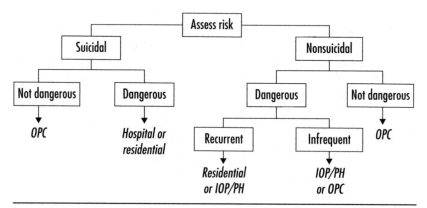

FIGURE 5–2. **Algorithm for selecting the level of care in response to self-endangering behaviors.**

Levels of care:
1. OPC=outpatient clinic/office practice
2. IOP/PH=intensive outpatient (>3 hours/week)/partial hospital (>10 hours/week)
3. Residential=structured living environments (e.g., halfway house)
4. Hospital

Source. Reprinted from Gunderson JG, Links P: *Handbook of Good Psychiatric Management for Borderline Personality Disorder.* Washington, DC, American Psychiatric Publishing, 2014, p. 41. Copyright © 2014 American Psychiatric Publishing. Used with permission.

standing through psychoeducation, taper unhelpful medications (polypharmacy), and approach difficult disclosures such as shameful failures or secrets. Teaching other ways of coping with distress and developing a crisis plan for the postdischarge period are the focus of inpatient admissions. The goal is discharge so patients can reenter life with increased tools and support to better manage self-destructive problems (Gunderson and Palmer 2019).

Involving Patients in Their Safety With Psychoeducation, Safety Planning, and Coping Skills

One way to approach suicidal behavior is to provide psychoeducation. Besides teaching how this behavior emerges, psychoeducation can also start a conversation about the feelings and thoughts teens with BPD have in these difficult moments, connecting symptoms to their real-life situations. In addition to increasing awareness, the objective is to help teens become more competent in managing themselves and using their social support network more appropriately. The clinician can say

> When you experience stressful interactions with someone
> close to you, such as trouble with your parents or an
> argument with a close friend, your emotions can get really
> intense. You may feel rejected and alone. Terrible thoughts
> may come across your mind, such as nobody cares, you are
> a loser, or you are bad. In the midst of this emotional
> turmoil, you can do things without thinking of the
> consequences as if to relieve yourself of something
> you feel inside. Does that make sense to you?

Patients should be partners in managing their safety. Sometimes, they expect you to tell them precisely what to do, but this can undermine their need to think for themselves and to develop self-agency. When you invite patients to say to you how you might help, they may not welcome this inquiry and may protest that "you are the expert." Furthermore, if there are acute safety concerns, clinicians may feel the urge to "take over" and to do things for their patients, especially when a young person is involved. Some patients hope for this. However, clinicians should keep the focus on agency as much as possible, even if it feels as if the stakes are too high. Educate patients that you will rely on them to be involved in their own rescue. Safety cannot depend solely on the availability of any one person, including you. Be honest by sharing that you can help more when you have the patient's perspective on what would help manage the situation. This conversation may need to be postponed to a scheduled session rather than in a crisis, when the patient may be under less pressure and can discuss your collaboration more constructively.

Developing a joint safety plan is a tool for adolescents to rely on as a first step and may help patients prevent self-harm. The safety plan outlines how patients can become more responsible for their own safety (Figure 5–3 and Table 5–4). The plan can start with identifying early warning signs (e.g., thought patterns, feelings, images, behaviors, urges) from previous crises. Then, clinicians and patients can work collaboratively to find different ways of coping with intense emotions and impulsivity (e.g., delaying action for 15 minutes, exercise, muscle relaxation, writing, distracting, interaction with a friend). Engage and motivate the patient by reviewing what has worked in the past or role-playing to teach these new skills. The construction of a "survival kit" with useful ways to self-soothe is another tool that can be helpful.

One way to introduce the use of coping skills is to say

> We can work together to develop new ways to cope with intense emotions and impulsivity. I think that increasing your autonomy to handle this will be helpful. I will help you learn how to do that over time. How does that sound?

Learning new skills can give hope and confidence, but it is important to stress that it requires training to become more competent, and these skills may not always work as expected. It is worth adding that these techniques are not a solution to the patient's issues but a tool for the patient to return to a more manageable level of distress. If none of this works, you can say to the adolescent

> Would it be possible to ask your parents to help you? They can offer you support. If this is not the case right now, I can work with them so that option is feasible in the future.
>
> Would it help to connect with someone? The interaction does not need to revolve around suicidality. In fact, it's better if it doesn't.
>
> Would it be useful to contact me or not? It's not that you can't ask me for help, but you don't want this to hinge on the likes of me.

Emphasize building a larger safety net of social supports as a key resource at difficult times. Patients with BPD may not know how to enlist support or elicit understanding without expressing their desperation. The key is to think collaboratively with the patient about what can be done to build a social network that can keep them more steady in general. Examining actions that are more prosocial and encouraging others to support this social connection process is key. With the teen, thoughtfully consider the effect that only expressing urgency and self-destructive worries may have on other people and on relationships. Such effects usually decrease interpersonal hypersensitivity.

SAFETY PLAN

Step 1: Warning Signs
- Feeling panicky and like I can't breathe; wanting to get out
- Wanting to take pills or drink

Step 2: Coping Using Distraction/Soothing Strategies
- Painting
- Petting my puppy

Step 3: Social Situations/People Who Can Help Distract Me
- My friends Patricia and Marie

Step 4: People I Can Ask for Help
(Note also if a person is unhelpful when you are in crisis.)
- My mom might be helpful
- Do not ask my boyfriend or sister for help during a crisis

Step 5: Professionals or Agencies I Can Contact During a Crisis
- National Suicide Prevention Lifeline: 1-800-273-8255
- List of others to be completed as homework

Step 6: Making the Environment Safer
- Lock my medications up so they are not readily available
- Cut my fake I.D. in half

FIGURE 5–3.   Safety planning example for adolescents.

The patient whose safety plan is shown here is a 16-year-old girl with a diagnosis of borderline personality disorder and a history of major depression. She has relatively minor self-harm behaviors and one recent low-lethality overdose attempt. Her self-harm behaviors are often precipitated by arguments with her on-again, off-again boyfriend or her sister.

Source.   Adapted from Gunderson and Links 2014, p. 152.

TABLE 5–4.   Coping skills

Think first!

Delay acting on impulses: chain analysis, writing, talking, counting to 10.

Introspection: "Try to understand what happened before you felt like this."

Write down the pros and cons of acting and not acting.

Recognize early warning signs (e.g., signs in the body and mental states) to prevent an escalation.

Avoid unhelpful coping strategies (e.g., isolating, substance use).

If it is not possible to think or to "slow down"[a]

Lower body temperature (e.g., cold water or ice packs on the cheeks for 30 seconds).

Exercise for 10–15 minutes.

Practice diaphragmatic breathing (e.g., breathe in for 4 seconds and out for 6–8 seconds).

Practice muscle relaxation exercises: tense and relax each muscle group, one at a time.

Other options

Distraction: play an instrument or a game, watch a comedy series or funny videos on the internet, do a puzzle.

Relaxation: listen to a guided meditation, take a break, stretch, go for a walk in a pleasant place.

Self-soothing: listen to music, look at pictures, eat a snack, drink a hot or cold nonalcoholic beverage, take a relaxing shower, imagine a happy and safe moment (past or future).

Creating meaning in a difficult situation: try to see things from a different and more positive perspective ("Make lemonade out of lemons"; "Every cloud has a silver lining").

Positive thinking: focus on positive thoughts (e.g., "I can face this"; "I will be all right").

For dissociative symptoms

Physical grounding skills: engage with salient external stimuli through the five senses (touch, taste, sound, smell, sight), such as putting one's feet on a cold floor.

Cognitive grounding skills: ask reorientation questions (e.g., "Where am I?" "What is the date?") or focus attention on concrete reality (e.g., "Name five objects in the room"; "Listen to the sounds of the surroundings"; "Count your breaths").

TABLE 5–4.   Coping skills *(continued)*

"Portable Survival Kit"

Include a safety plan and objects that can be helpful outside the home.

Apps

Use apps that can help coach teenagers with coping skills and safety planning. Choose one that you know and teach the teen how to use it. However, this should not preclude active learning on the part of the patient.

---

[a]If there is any physical comorbidity (e.g., cold temperature and intense exercise in teenagers with heart disease) that raises caution about the use of any of these skills, a physician should be consulted.

Source.   Bateman and Fonagy 2016; Gunderson and Links 2014; Rathus and Miller 2014.

Help the patient develop healthy socialization with friends, peers, and family in a way that is expected during their development:

> Although I can help you manage these behaviors, to diminish their cause, we also need to help you find better social supports—people to help you with those situations.

Parents should also be partners in their teen's safety and allies in regulating the teen's emotions in times of crisis (Figure 5–4). In some families, the relationships are tense, but the role of the parents should be explored because they are the first and foremost individuals responsible for keeping the teen safe. Therefore, they should be included in the crisis plan whenever possible and should work to limit access to lethal means, if necessary. Parents may need help in putting the teen's self-harm or suicidality in context so that they can know how to be helpful. Teaching adolescents how to ask their parents or others for help is important, as well as establishing a plan for parents for which the adolescent participates in constructing. If this is clearly not possible, it is useful to search for another adult (e.g., another family member) to play this role to assist the patient.

Clinician Limitations

Performing a suicide risk assessment is not magically forecasting whether a patient will complete suicide. We cannot precisely predict suicidality (Black et al. 2004) or read teenagers' minds. Nor can we undo the consequences after self-harm occurs. It is essential to be frank about what you can and cannot do (limits) and to ask patients to communicate when they

PARENT COPING PLAN

→ 1: Possible Triggers
- Final exams
- Fight with younger brother

→ 2: Warning Signs
- Sudden mood changes
- Dysregulated eating
- Troubled sleeping

→ 3: Remember My Emotional Management
- Breathe in and out
- Remember: "I love my son"
- Notice how I am feeling
- Allow myself to be hurt

→ 4: Helpful Attitudes Toward My Teen
- Try to listen & understand what happened ("be curious")
- Keep my voice down and avoid sarcasm
- Communicate my understanding in a nonjudgmental manner
- Support (example: "I am here to help you")
- Help in following the safety plan collaboratively
- Choose the timing of discussions about other subjects.

→ 5: Unhelpful Attitudes Toward My Teen
- Panic
- Overreacting and arguing
- Judgments: blame, rights, and wrongs
- Jumping to conclusions
- Giving in to angry outbursts

→ 6: If nothing else helps and there is an emergency
- Professional help

FIGURE 5–4. **Coping plan example for parents.**

Lucy is the mother of Michael, a 14-year-old teenager who has BPD. He has a history of episodes with angry outbursts and impulsivity, followed by intense sadness and shame triggered by interpersonal and academic stress. The clinician has built a coping plan collaboratively with Lucy, keeping in mind Michael's history and his interactions with her in times of distress. Past helpful and unhelpful attitudes toward Michael were blended with new coping skills for the family.

are in danger. Get their feedback to check if they understood your guidance. Do not act as if you are omniscient or omnipotent. It is also not realistic for the patient or family to expect your unlimited availability (see section "Intersession Availability" in Chapter 4).

Involving Colleagues

Discussing cases with colleagues helps clinicians regulate their own emotions and see different alternatives when dealing with a difficult situation. Supervision by peers or experts can decrease your emotional burden. It also provides a source of perspective and consultation, which reflects an accepted approach to risk management and liability (see Table 5–3).

Involving the Family and School

Involving parents or guardians in safety planning (e.g., coping skills to buffer the crisis) may decrease family distress and benefit patients (Flynn et al. 2017). Parents' difficulties in managing their fearful and angry responses can aggravate an already overwhelming problem for adolescents (Buckholdt et al. 2014). Normalizing and supporting these challenges for parents can enlist their collaboration, which will be needed to allow you to instruct them on what they can do better. Families need and often want help with this and will be receptive to support through family groups and treatment referrals.

Involving school professionals allows you to facilitate problem solving that cannot otherwise be organized. You can provide psychoeducation and guidelines on how to adapt to and work with an adolescent with BPD. Family guidelines may be adapted for schools (see Appendix D, "Guidelines for Families"). This may increase school attendance and provide additional support for the teenager. Schools vary widely in how they are prepared to deal with mental health disorders. Some may need more education and knowledge. Reintegration into environments where the adolescent is socially connected and engaged in purposeful activities can be a source of a needed longer-term stabilization.

Aftermath of Self-Endangering Behaviors

Nonsuicidal Self-Injury or Nonfatal Suicide Attempts

Complete an Interpersonal Chain Analysis

Detailing the events that precipitated self-injurious behavior is an exercise with many functions (see Chapter 4, Figure 4–2). Besides identifying the interpersonal precipitants, an interpersonal chain analysis offers the lesson that emotions do not come out of the blue. Adolescents will then learn to better identify their thoughts and feelings, which has utility beyond the management of safety. You can ask patients in a noncritical manner what they think the impact of their self-destructive behavior on others was. Understanding transactions that occur and connecting actions with feelings or thoughts help clarify how social exchange works. Specifically, knowing that they may have scared someone with their suicidality, causing a reaction of withdrawal or anger, can help adolescents see a less personalized explanation (e.g., suicidality causes anxiety) that can replace the reflexive interpretation of being "bad" or "toxic" as the cause. Drawing or writing a time line of the analysis helps teens better visualize what happened.

Some patients may resist doing this exercise because it will expose them to a feared inner state or because they feel shame about it. They may use the same familiar dysfunctional coping skills (e.g., suppressing, avoiding, "acting out"), but you can validate their difficulty and help them accept their emotional reactions (Andrewes et al. 2017). Proper emotional management in the here and now shows that they will not necessarily lose control. Teaching ways of coping within sessions is also an opportunity to show how handling crises differently is doable.

Discuss the Interpersonal Stressor and Interpret What Provided Relief

When exploring the interpersonal context that prompted self-injurious behavior, look for feelings of rejection, abandonment, and loneliness, as well as shame, self-criticism, and low self-esteem. In analyzing the consequences of self-destructive behavior, discuss what provided relief (e.g., did the patient feel cared for, or was the psychological pain so intense that they needed to distract?). Underscoring interpersonal hypersensitivity is a helpful way for patients to accept this vulnerability and to better predict their reactions in social interactions.

Anticipate Future Safety Issues

After exploring the past chain of events, it is vital to think about possible upcoming events, develop a new safety plan, and consider new learning from the crisis at hand. When elaborating on the new plan, it is essential to discuss earlier signs of distress, to teach different ways of coping, and to involve the patient in generating various alternatives in problem-solving ("Thinking about this now, was there anything you could have done?"). Be transparent in telling the effect on you ("I was preoccupied") and then emphasize the unfeasibility of depending on you to be in charge of providing safety during crisis (see Figure 5–3).

Promote School Reintegration

Some patients may have difficulty returning to school. They will face teachers and colleagues after a hospitalization, feel shame, and worry about the judgment of their peers. In addition, they might have a lot of academic work to catch up on, which would be overwhelming for anyone. Schools with more structured time management and learning support can provide a constructive environment for these patients (Kasen et al. 2009). In addition, it is very important to construct a plan of reintegration involving the mental health team, parents, and school to avoid rehospitalization and dropout.

Staff at schools will be reasonably worried about managing the patient's self-destructive problems. Providing psychoeducation and clarifying roles within the scope of the job everyone has can settle anxieties. Be clear that your job is working with the patient within their psychiatric care to find alternative ways to manage distress other than suicidality and self-harm, whereas theirs is to foster a learning environment for the patient to build a life that offers structure, activity, and community for rehabilitation. You may need to educate school staff about the limitations of psychiatric hospitalization, as well as the need for the student to take leave from school repeatedly as a solution to their stress intolerance. Offer to assist the staff and convey that you and they work as a team. Here are some useful guidelines (Tougas et al. 2019):

- Mental health team: Schedule predictable regular follow-ups, provide psychoeducation, communicate with parents and the school for individualized plans, teach coping and social skills to the patient.
- School: Accommodate the patient's needs, deal effectively with crises, set realistic goals regarding school performance, have one member of staff (e.g., principal, adviser) aware of the teen's history and helping him or individually, be informed by the mental health team regarding the patient's condition and treatment (via a document or a meeting).
- Parents: Learn about available public and private resources, support the teen in reintegration, communicate with the school regarding their child's disorder.

If all efforts to reintegrate with additional support are unsuccessful, then other alternatives (e.g., specialist advice, changing schools or homeschooling) can be sought. When possible, help the student adapt and effectively gain help where they are because transitions to new environments can also be destabilizing when the student is in crisis.

Death From Suicide

Suicides in adolescents are devastating for families and clinicians. The ambivalence and impulsivity of individuals with BPD usually make us think about what factors could have delayed or prevented the final act, especially in young individuals whom we hoped to help with early intervention. The first task is to inform the authorities, clinical staff, and family. Then, clinicians should carefully document the last interaction with the patient. It is important to meet with the family, offer your condolences, and listen. Suggest referrals, if needed. On the clinician's part, it is important to seek out colleagues and supervisors to discuss the experience because deaths from suicide can be quite traumatic (Sakinofsky 2007), especially for trainees. Acceptance that not all suicides can be prevented, remembering that it is an inherent risk in our profession, and validation of this painful experience may help. Having formal meetings with clinical staff, acknowledging the stress of the event, and going through a psychological autopsy after the shock passes will help clinicians learn from the event (Al-Mateen et al. 2018).

Common Problems

Your Patient's Suicidality Is Not Diminishing

Suicidal behavior may wax and wane, mainly in times of interpersonal stress. However, it is expected that such behaviors will decrease over time. If suicidal behaviors persist, seek consultation. The first crucial question is, "Am I missing something here?" A collaborative conversation with the patient can be made carefully without blaming them for the situation. Highlighting the limitations you may have as a sole provider for helping diminish suicidality names a clinical problem to be addressed. Expanding the support safety net may require another clinician to perform a complementary role (see Chapter 7, "Multimodal Treatments").

Examine which factors may be sustaining suicidality (i.e., motives and consequences of these behaviors). Investigate the family environment (including use of social services support, if available and necessary), identify potential blind spots (e.g., abuse, concerns about sexual orientation, fantasies about suicide), examine the therapeutic relationship (e.g., emotions toward treatment, activity in the treatment), and consider why your interventions are not working. For instance, avoidance of real life as well as fear of losing support might be maintaining a regressed, dependent state in the patient. Sometimes, other options (i.e., having a life) seem too unreal or too frightening. Clinicians should validate the feelings patients can express, without certainty or rigidity about what needs to happen, and wonder with the patient what other ways there are to manage distress and other feelings that are identified.

If suicidality continues even after your interventions, seeking out a more specialized treatment (e.g., dialectical behavior therapy for adolescents, mentalization-based treatment for adolescents, residential level of care) might be an option where available, although that may be rarely the case. In the absence of this option, other available resources can be considered actively with the patient and the family. If no other preferred alternatives exist, share your view of what would be needed to make the treatment with you more effective. Broad consideration of options can in and of itself be a helpful exercise for the patient and family in "thinking first" and making a rational choice about the path they take because they will be informed by you to do so.

Challenges arise when the focus is shifted from symptomatic remission to other aspects of the patient's life. After finding the source of mental anguish that makes a patient suicidal, you can accept it, validate it, and in parallel work with a person-centered approach, helping the patient progress through their values and goals, trying to reinforce more adaptive behavior and increase the quality of life (Hennings 2020). This way, it is possible for patients to build a more positive narrative of themselves over time.

The Patient Seeks Hospitalization for Suicidality, but You Do Not Think They Are in Danger

If there is not a shared agreement regarding how you and the patient manage suicidality and you do not hospitalize the patient, the risk is increased significantly. One way of dealing with this is the principle of "false submission" (Gunderson 2008; Gunderson and Links 2014, p. 44):

> I'm willing to hospitalize you, but I am not sure if it will help. I will do this because I fear you will become more suicidal if I don't. Am I right about that? We would both be better off if we could find another way to deal with this.

This makes the dilemma explicit and involves the patient as a collaborator in exploring why they want to go to an inpatient unit (e.g., it means you care or it is a solution to the problem) and helps clinicians discuss the pros and cons. This statement also allows the clinician to express a conflict rather than focus solely on action. Hospitalizing a patient can be important for safety, but it may reinforce avoidant strategies. About 28% of suicidal adolescents are rehospitalized within 6 months of index admission (Yen et al. 2014). Discussing the difficulty of finding other ways to manage as a dilemma you share together allows you to candidly address the issue and discuss alternatives.

Your Patient With Dangerous Self-Harming Behavior Refuses to Give You Permission to Contact Significant Others

Safety takes precedence over confidentiality. Clinicians need to involve significant others in safety management, even if patients resist. There may be different reasons for the resistance, or it can be due to "all good or all bad" cognition. This will need to be discussed with the adolescent in a way that is collaborative rather than authoritative, as in the following series of questions asked by a clinician dealing with refusal from a patient.

Setting Common Goals

Adolescents might refuse permission for the clinician to talk with their parents for several reasons. However, most of them will accept help in relationship management to decrease conflicts and problems at home. Even if the patient feels hopeless (e.g., because no practitioner has been able to help them in this regard), the clinician might say the following:

> I understand that you don't want me to contact or talk with your parents. And I am not really sure why. Is there any trouble in your relationship or at home that I can help you with?

Concerns About Confidentiality From Clinician

Another common situation is that teens might be cautious of disclosing sensitive subjects (e.g., normative sexual experiences) to their parents or think that their parents are too controlling. In these situations, the clinician can say the following:

> Is there anything that you are afraid of disclosing to your parents? I am worried about your safety, and that is what I want to talk about.

Sharing the Dilemma

In more challenging situations, disclosing the dilemma that the clinician is facing may be useful if applied carefully. It is essential to monitor the patient's reaction and to convey honesty and transparency, not the idea of a threat. The clinician can share the dilemma this way:

> If I take the path of not talking with your parents, you will feel more comfortable now, and we will not argue. In that sense, it is easier for me. But I will be very concerned about your safety and who can help you outside. I don't want you to be without any help in these situations. If I take the other path, by talking with your parents, you may be angry at me. Teaching your parents better ways to support you may help, but our collaborative relationship will be undermined. Then, I fear you will not trust me. How can we work on that?

Clinicians have the legal right to contact family members, even when there is no longer suicidal ideation, because these behaviors can recur in times of stress, and some patients may underestimate the dangerousness of their impulsive acts. Involving significant people in the patient's life is also useful for monitoring changes in risk, for gathering helpful information (environment and facts not disclosed), for safety planning, and during the postdischarge period when the suicide risk is higher.

Your Patient Will Not Agree to Take Suicide "Off the Table"

Sometimes, patients may not agree to work on decreasing their suicidality. It is important to note that chronic suicidality is different in many ways (e.g., function, symptoms) from acute crisis (Weinberg and Maltsberger 2007). Hospitalization has limited therapeutic impact in treating this kind of suicidality. Some patients may regulate themselves with suicidal thoughts that can also be a way to exert control (Hennings 2020). These patients have suicidal ideation, but they are not acutely dysregulated, intending to act on their thoughts immediately (Maltsberger et al. 2010).

If clinicians agree to work with these patients, they need to be able to tolerate this suicidality, and the family must accept the possibility of suicide. In these cases, it is necessary to ask for a second opinion from another clinician to assess whether a safer alternative can be arranged. These measures aid liability management (Kernberg 1993). The same principles of working in areas of a patient's life other than suicidality can be helpful, as stated in the subsection "Your Patient's Suicidality Is Not Diminishing."

Your Patient Will Not Agree to Decrease Self-Harm Behaviors

Self-harm is not the primary target of GPM, although it is expected to diminish over time. Chain analyses may help clinicians tailor alternative coping strategies (Nock 2010). For example, if the primary function is emotion regulation (reducing anxiety or dissociation), teach emotion and impulsivity management tools and grounding techniques. If it is social regulation (seeking help or escape from a difficult situation), or if self-harm is used to communicate distress, thinking with patients about how they can communicate more directly will be helpful. You may increase motivation to change, stating the pros and cons of the self-harming and evaluating how compatible self-destructive action is with the patient's

Chapter 6

Pharmacotherapy and Comorbidity

Carl Fleisher, M.D.

Sara Rose Masland, Ph.D.

General Principles

Be Active, Not Reactive

We advise a planned, "less is more" approach to pharmacotherapy for adolescents with borderline personality disorder (BPD; Bozzatello et al. 2020). Avoid prescribing medication and prevent the need for it through robust psychosocial intervention. Good psychiatric management (GPM) reminds prescribers to ground themselves according to usual standards of care, combined with knowledge about current research on the efficacy of pharmacological interventions for BPD and its common comorbidities. When prescribing is unavoidable, use medication at low doses for short periods of time. The structure, flexibility, and optimism of such an approach can provide a boost to patients, which in turn can enhance their alliance and collaboration. This approach underscores our belief that the relationship with the prescriber is more important than whether medication is prescribed, or which one (Gunderson and Choi-Kain 2018). Put another way, clinicians need not encourage, nor expect much from, pharmacotherapy (Biskin 2013). GPM's approach is based on the patient's current state (for details, see Figure 6–1). Possible states include the following:

- *Acutely, but not severely, distressed* patients must learn to use coping skills. In acute distress, the benefit of any medication is typically small. Medication could engender either a negative or a positive placebo effect.
- *If a patient requests medication* but is not severely distressed, be cautious—reactive prescribing may reinforce the patient's lack of agency in coping with challenges. Selective serotonin reuptake inhibitors (SSRIs) can be considered because they pose little risk yet may offer modest benefit.
- *For patients who are severely distressed*, prescribers can suggest medication. If they or their parents decline, however, watchful waiting is reasonable.
- *Avoid polypharmacy*. Explain in advance a policy that if stated goals are not achieved, the medication will be discontinued before beginning any other one. (In situations of severe distress, a cross-taper may be appropriate.)

Avoid a Dichotomous View

Patients or parents may hold a dichotomous view, that is, medication either works or it doesn't, the patient is depressed or is not. Avoid colluding with such a perspective. Share your healthy skepticism based on research, emphasize potential downsides of medication, and offer hope that situations will pass with or without a prescription. Remind patients and their families just how broad the array of factors is that influence them on a given day: peers, school, sexuality and gender, sleep, social media and other screen use, family (vis-à-vis privacy or independence), and more.

Consider Stage of Illness

The pathology of BPD is fluid in adolescence. Symptoms of BPD may wax and wane as development progresses or even improve as adolescence

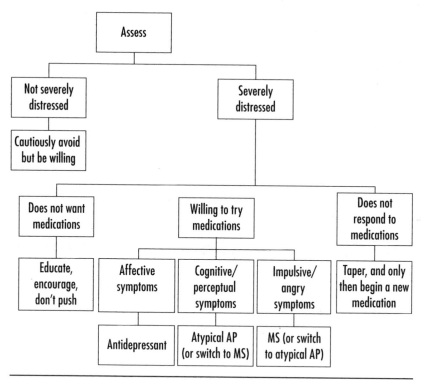

FIGURE 6–1. **Algorithm for medication choice.**

AP=antipsychotic; MS=mood stabilizer.

Source. Adapted from Gunderson and Links 2014, p. 50.

ends. Notably, adolescents with subthreshold BPD (DSM-5 Cluster B traits)—or simply unrecognized full-threshold BPD—may suffer significant impairment and distress (American Psychiatric Association 2013; Sharp and Wall 2018; Thompson et al. 2019b). In turn, clinicians may find themselves asked to prescribe for an adolescent at any point in the course of BPD: emerging, threshold, relapsing, or convalescent. We encourage clinicians to consider each adolescent's trajectory when evaluating the role of medication for a given symptom or situation.

Building an Alliance

The prescriber must build two strong alliances: with the adolescent and with the parent or guardian(s). Each person involved in treatment has their own set of knowledge, expectations, reservations about medication, and observations of mood and behavior. These must be respected and accounted for in some way to earn trust. When prescribers state their own expectations, that helps to shape realistic expectations for patients and families, too.

Provide Psychoeducation

Psychoeducation is therapeutic; it may even preclude the need for medication (Ridolfi et al. 2019). Encourage optimism about the patient's prognosis despite the absence of a clear role for medication (Soloff and Chiappetta 2019). Be open about the shortcomings of current research (Biskin 2013). Emphasize that medication is adjunctive at best and can cause more harm than good (Ingenhoven and Duivenvoorden 2011). Be aware that using medication may communicate an expectation that patients cannot cope with stress on their own.

Pay Concerned, Thoughtful Attention

Crises grab everyone's attention. Yet too often, patients or families do not respond to less dramatic events that nonetheless contribute to said crises. Prescribers can express empathy about crises and also bring families' attention to subtler problems. Doing so helps to model reflection, as well as promotes learning and coping.

Emphasize Need for Collaboration

Successful treatment requires collaboration. Providers, parents, and the adolescent involved must work as a team to navigate when to prescribe, how much, and for how long. Establish metrics of change—things that can be detected, described, and demonstrated. Encourage tracking of mood, school tardiness, hours of sleep, or other relevant symptoms (Firth et al. 2017; Rickard et al. 2016). When such measurement demonstrates the usefulness, or uselessness, of medication, the team can weigh that against any side effects that occur. Tracking change may provide added benefits: it can stimulate agency, self-awareness, and appreciation of nuance.

When prescribing, a collaborative process should yield clear expectations. Prescribing should be related to treatment goals; "feeling better" is not enough by itself. Consensus around the goals of medication use is ideal. However, it is also common for adolescents and their parent(s) to envision different goals. It is more important that each understand the other's goal than that they agree. Discussions should preview discontinuation of medication. Without predetermined duration of use and milestones for discontinuation, a medication initiated during a crisis may become a long-term crutch of uncertain benefit. Although you need not delay starting medication in a true crisis, offering frequent appointments (every 1–2 weeks) may both alleviate the pressure for an immediate intervention and allow adequate time to discuss each of the parameters involved in thoughtful prescribing.

Elicit Negative Expectations

Inquire about negative attitudes, reservations, and anecdotes of bad experiences lest they derail your interventions. Seeking to understand negative attitudes will earn trust; grasping them fully might uncover opportunities to avoid or ameliorate problems. Conversely, some negative attitudes about medication may be a boon. At times when medication is requested but the prescriber recommends against using it, the prescriber can emphasize any preexisting reservations a patient or family member has had about pharmacological intervention.

Selecting Medications

General Comments

For all medications, little research guides dosing (e.g., Bozzatello et al. 2020; Ingenhoven and Duivenvoorden 2011). Table 6–1 summarizes the limitations of current knowledge. Certain classes of medication may be more effective at addressing certain symptoms of BPD (Abraham and Calabrese 2008; Mercer et al. 2009; Vita et al. 2011); see summary in Table 6–2. Patients with BPD may experience improvement at unexpectedly low doses of medication or may be more vulnerable to adverse effects—or at least they may view themselves that way. To account for these possibilities, we recommend starting any medication at a low, subtherapeutic dose. Likewise, if titrating, do so more gradually than you would in the absence of BPD. Prescribers may still aim to reach typical, "therapeutic" doses of a given medication, but because existing data already provide only weak support for typical dosing, the use of supratherapeutic doses is not recommended. Polypharmacy is excessively common among adolescents with BPD (Cailhol et al. 2013). However, there is no identifiable benefit to this approach; hence, it should be avoided (Biskin 2013; Bozzatello et al. 2020).

Interactions With Alcohol or Marijuana (and Possibly Other Drugs)

Any foray into prescribing to adolescents, particularly those with BPD, requires a discussion of interactions with alcohol and drugs. This includes

---

TABLE 6–1. Current status of pharmacotherapy for borderline personality disorder

---

Approximately 50 randomized controlled trials have been conducted (antipsychotics > mood stabilizers > others > antidepressants).

Trials typically had small sample sizes (average $N=40$), variable outcome measures, and limited duration (4–12 weeks).

Funding and generalizability of research have been hampered by fears of liability for violence, suicide, or self-harm.

No medication is uniformly helpful, and none has been approved by a governmental agency (FDA or EMA).

Medication does not address the interpersonal hypersensitivity core of BPD.

Polypharmacy is of unproven benefit, is often inversely related to improvement, and is associated with adverse effects.

National guidelines differ from each other in regard to whether medication is recommended, under what circumstances, of what type, and for how long.

Note. BPD=borderline personality disorder; EMA=European Medicines Agency.

Source. Adapted from Gunderson and Links 2014, p. 49.

---

drug-medication interactions, such as with cocaine and stimulants, and also drug-medication-judgment interactions, such as the potential for unsafe decision-making when drinking alcohol, which has more potent effects while taking SSRIs. Have this discussion with adolescents and their parent(s) or guardian(s) together. A separate, more detailed conversation with the adolescent also may be warranted.

Cannabis use—either the whole plant or cannabidiol—is increasingly common among adolescents (Johnston et al. 2018). Insisting that they stop using would be fruitless and would undermine their agency. Instead, meet adolescents where they are. Motivational interviewing techniques are invaluable here: be curious ("How do you think about your marijuana use?") and respect the rewarding aspects of use ("Tell me what you enjoy about using marijuana") but encourage patients to take a balanced view by considering drawbacks of use ("Is there anything you don't like about using marijuana?"). Provide patients with information and resources from which they can educate themselves (Gobbi et al. 2019). Offer to negotiate about use, without judgment, when appropriate ("Is there any way

TABLE 6–2. Symptom targets and medication types

	Mood instability	Depression	Anxiety	Anger	Impulsivity	Cognitive/perceptual
Antidepressants	+	±	+	+	±	−/?
Mood stabilizers	+	+	++	++	+/++	−/?
Antipsychotics	+	−	−/?	++	±	++

Note. ++=helpful; +=modestly helpful; ?=uncertain; −=not helpful.

Source. Adapted from Gunderson and Links 2014, p. 51; Mercer et al. 2009; Silk and Feurino 2012.

to interest you in cutting back?"), or try using shaping (i.e., give a small reward for any action in the direction of eventually decreasing use).

Antidepressants

SSRIs are prescribed more commonly than other types of antidepressants. This predominance of SSRI prescribing presumably stems both from the fact that they are approved by the FDA for use in pediatric populations and because of their relatively mild side-effect profile. Nonetheless, what research there is—almost exclusively in adults—shows that SSRIs have limited benefit for depression or anxiety comorbid with BPD (Ingenhoven et al. 2010; Vita et al. 2011). When SSRIs are ineffective, reuptake inhibitors of serotonin and norepinephrine, or of dopamine, also may be tried. In general, there are mixed data supporting antidepressants' effectiveness in treating depression and impulsivity but primarily positive results supporting their amelioration of anxiety, anger, and mood instability (Bozzatello et al. 2020; Ingenhoven and Duivenvoorden 2011; Mercer et al. 2009; Nosè et al. 2006; Vita et al. 2011). Tricyclic antidepressants and monoamine oxidase inhibitors are relatively contraindicated in adolescents because of their lethality in overdose, especially when considering the impulsivity of some adolescents with BPD (Bozzatello et al. 2020).

SSRIs are not approved to treat BPD itself. They also are subject to a black box warning issued by the FDA regarding possible increases in suicidality (U.S. Food and Drug Administration 2018). (A parallel warning has been issued by the European Medicines Agency.) This warning must and should be discussed as part of the informed consent process (Spielmans et al. 2020). Nonetheless, prescribers may want to emphasize the black box warning when patients are seeking medication that is not clinically indicated. On the other hand, prescribers may decide to deemphasize the warning when an SSRI trial seems justified but the patient or parents are hesitant to proceed.

Mood Stabilizers

Limited data, available only in adults, support the effectiveness of mood stabilizers for anger, mood, anxiety, and impulsivity in BPD (Abraham and Calabrese 2008; Bozzatello et al. 2020; Mercer et al. 2009). However, many mood stabilizers are recognized teratogens. Side effects such as cognitive dulling and photosensitivity are additional drawbacks. Lamotrigine may be effective for some patients (Reich et al. 2009; Tritt et al. 2005), but it is neither cost-effective on a broad scale nor superior to placebo (Crawford et al. 2018). The liabilities of lamotrigine's rare but serious side effects, especially with nonadherence to regular dosing, should be considered. All other mood stabilizers besides lamotrigine require laboratory testing, both at baseline and periodically throughout treatment. If prescribing, use typical doses.

Antipsychotics

Antipsychotic medications may be helpful in treating anger, impulsivity, or psychotic experiences and improving cognitive or perceptual deficits (Bridler et al. 2015; Nosè et al. 2006; Vita et al. 2011). Use the lowest possible doses. Aripiprazole, ziprasidone, and possibly risperidone are less likely than quetiapine or olanzapine to cause rapid, significant weight gain (Stigler et al. 2004). Compliance with the recommended schedule of monitoring weight, metabolism (with blood tests), and involuntary movements is essential (Ho et al. 2011).

Anxiolytics

For adolescents with BPD, there is a strong relative contraindication to benzodiazepine use (Bridler et al. 2015). When use is chronic—whether initiated by the prescriber or inherited from a prior prescriber—it is critical to be sure the patient and family are aware of the possibility of life-threatening withdrawal.

Medications for ADHD

ADHD comorbid with BPD warrants typical treatment, as one would do in the absence of BPD (Golubchik et al. 2008). Give consideration to stimulants, nonstimulants, and trigeminal nerve stimulation. Stimulant medication might be particularly helpful in addressing impulsivity shared between ADHD and BPD. Caution is advised, of course, for patients with significant substance misuse. Notably, adolescents misusing "uppers" (e.g., cocaine, amphetamines) may be attempting to self-medicate inattention rather than using for emotion regulation. Patients who self-medicate may be able to curtail misuse when offered appropriate supervised treatment.

Other Medications

Recent review of the literature on pharmacotherapy for BPD suggests (Bozzatello et al. 2020) the following:

- (Es)ketamine—no data support its use.

- Naltrexone—may offer benefit for excessive alcohol use or behavioral addictions. Naltrexone may offer limited benefit for self-harm, with few side effects, on the basis of the rationale that self-harm is compulsive in nature.
- Clonidine—highly sedating; hence may reduce insomnia. Studies have also shown modest impact on self-harm and on dissociation.
- Omega-3 fatty acids—may have generic benefits; harmless. In BPD, it may reduce depression, anger, impulsivity, and self-harm (Amminger et al. 2013).
- Somatic therapies:
  - Transcranial magnetic stimulation—shows promising effects in adolescents with refractory depression, but no data clarify whether comorbid BPD impacts rate of response.
  - Electroconvulsive therapy (ECT)—in adults, comorbid BPD clearly reduces response rates and leads to higher likelihood of relapse. Patients with BPD also tend to have capricious reactions to ECT or become inappropriately attached to ECT (Rasmussen 2015). There are no data in adolescents. This treatment should be pursued rarely, if ever.

Comorbidities

Selecting Primary Diagnostic Target

Comorbidity with BPD is the rule rather than the exception. Indeed, having BPD exacerbates illnesses such as substance use disorder, and substance use disorders may impede the otherwise gradual decline in BPD psychopathology (Bornovalova et al. 2018). Hence, the clinician's task often is to assess for both BPD and comorbid diagnoses. Complicating matters is the fact that adolescents with BPD commonly present with symptoms of a comorbid illness rather than with symptoms of BPD. This may be because of stigma or lack of recognition of the underlying illness. Telltale—although not diagnostic—indications of underlying BPD include coexisting internalizing and externalizing disorders, polypharmacy, "refractory" illness, history of needing a higher level of care, or a history of multiple (5–10 or more) medication trials.

When comorbid diagnoses are present, clinicians are faced with the task of deciding which disorder to focus on treating. Longitudinal research (Grilo et al. 2010; Gunderson et al. 2004) suggests that for some comorbid diagnoses, improvement is unlikely (or recurrence is more likely) unless BPD is treated. In other words, BPD is the primary illness (Table 6–3). This group includes major depression, anxiety, and narcissistic personality disorder. In addition, for certain comorbid diagnoses that require distinct treatment (e.g., obsessive-compulsive disorder), we recommend an initial focus on BPD in order to stabilize the patient's ability to engage in treatment at all.

Other comorbid diagnoses will not improve unless treated directly (Grilo et al. 2010; Gunderson et al. 2004). These include ADHD (see earlier subsection "Medications for ADHD"), mania, and anorexia nervosa; their symptoms may preclude either participation in treatment, motivation, rational cognition, or academic achievement and learning. BPD is secondary when treating these disorders (Table 6–4). Notably, children with preexisting ADHD who suffer maltreatment may be even more likely to develop BPD (Calvo et al. 2020). When addressing ADHD, take care to follow the standard of care, including tracking symptoms with validated parent and teacher rating scales (e.g., Weibel et al. 2018).

Determining Priority for Treatment

With some comorbid diagnoses, establishing treatment priority requires clinical judgment. Included in this group are PTSD, substance use disorders, bulimia nervosa, and bipolar II disorder. The severity of these illnesses varies, and patients may vary in their openness to addressing certain symptoms, so the priorities and intensity of treatment must also change.

Concerning PTSD, for example, Shea et al. (2004) found that improvement in BPD symptoms predicted PTSD remission. Keuroghlian and colleagues (2015) found that PTSD significantly impacted the course of BPD, predicting BPD relapse. Findings are also mixed as to whether BPD treatment can reduce PTSD symptoms. Although some studies of BPD treatment alone have not reported success in improving co-occurring PTSD (Harned et al. 2008), others show equal effectiveness in treating patients with BPD, with and without PTSD (Boritz et al. 2016; Gratz et al. 2020; Harned et al. 2010; Masland et al. 2019). Evidence-based treatments targeting BPD and PTSD concurrently have been developed and have shown greater improvements in both BPD and PTSD symptoms (Bohus et al. 2013, 2020; Harned et al. 2014), as well as functional outcomes (Harned et al. 2018), compared with standard BPD or PTSD treatments.

With clinically significant substance use, concurrent treatment might be warranted, and at times, the patient might enter a detoxification facility or begin a long period of sobriety. Particularly when it comes to substance use, parents' assistance is often helpful because many adolescents struggle to limit use on their own. Clinicians can work with parents to establish con-

TABLE 6–3. **Borderline personality disorder (BPD) comorbidity in which BPD is primary**

Disorder	Comorbidity with BPD (%)[a]	% BPD in this disorder[a]	Notes[b]
Mood and anxiety disorders			
Major depressive disorder	80	20	Depression will remit if BPD does.
Anxiety	60	7–21	Anxiety will remit if BPD does. Address anxiety as coprimary if school refusal is present.
Bipolar I disorder (euthymic or depressed)	12	15	Course is independent of BPD.
Bipolar II disorder	8	40	Course is independent of BPD.
PTSD[c]	32–47	8–29	
Prepubertal onset/ complex			BPD is primary if patient is not too vigilant to attach or be challenged.
Adolescent onset			If able to use BPD treatment, treating BPD will help with PTSD, especially if patient is older adolescent (16–18 years).
Substance use			
Intermittent or binge use	Unknown	Unknown	When substance use is infrequent and exclusively serves to regulate emotions, it will remit if BPD does.

TABLE 6–3. **Borderline personality disorder (BPD) comorbidity in which BPD is primary *(continued)***

Disorder	Comorbidity with BPD (%)[a]	% BPD in this disorder[a]	Notes[b]
Substance use *(continued)*			
Substance use disorder	50	10–20	Sobriety for 3–6 months is ideal. However, consistent sobriety may require BPD treatment
Personality disorder			
Antisocial personality disorder	14–15	21	BPD is primary if treatment is not for secondary gain.
Narcissistic personality disorder (NPD)	8–39	37	Treating BPD may make NPD treatment more effective.
Eating disorder	20	20	
Bulimia nervosa	13	28	Treat BPD if patient is medically stable.
Sleep problems	17–45	Unknown	Start with sleep hygiene, including technology use; problems with sleep will remit if BPD does.

[a]These are adult data from Asaad et al. 2002; Grant et al. 2008; McGlashan et al. 2000; Plante et al. 2009; Sansone et al. 2004; Zanarini et al. 2004.

[b]This reasoning is based on longitudinal research summarized by Gunderson et al. 2004, 2014, 2018; Keuroghlian et al. 2015; Lee et al. 2015; Pennay et al. 2011.

[c]PTSD may be primary or secondary, depending on severity and on patient characteristics. See text for details.

Source. Adapted from Gunderson and Links 2014, p. 53.

TABLE 6–4.   Borderline personality disorder (BPD) comorbidity in which BPD is secondary

Disorder	% in BPD[a]	% BPD in this disorder[a]	Notes[b]
ADHD	38	14	Interferes with academic achievement unless treated. ADHD has a distinct pathophysiology. Offer typical treatment. Use caution when substance use disorder is present.
Bipolar I disorder	12	15	
During manic episodes			Patient may be unable to use BPD therapy because of irrational cognition.
PTSD[c]	32–47	8–29	
Prepubertal/ complex			BPD is secondary if patient is too vigilant to attach or be challenged.
Adolescent onset			BPD is secondary if PTSD symptoms interfere with treatment for BPD.
Substance use	50	10–20	Active use interferes with motivation for treatment. Sobriety for 3–6 months is ideal. Consistent sobriety may require focus on BPD.

TABLE 6–4. **Borderline personality disorder (BPD) comorbidity in which BPD is secondary** *(continued)*

Disorder	% in BPD[a]	% BPD in this disorder[a]	Notes[b]
Antisocial personality disorder	14–15	21	BPD is secondary if treatment is for secondary gain
Eating disorder	20	20	
Anorexia nervosa	7	25	Treat the eating disorder first if patient is medically unstable or is unable to be present for or participate in BPD treatment.
Bulimia nervosa	13	28	Treat the eating disorder first if patient is medically unstable.

[a]These are adult data from Ferrer et al. 2010; Grant et al. 2008; McGlashan et al. 2000; Miller et al. 2008; Sansone et al. 2004.

[b]This reasoning is based on longitudinal research summarized by Gunderson et al. 2004, 2014, 2018; Keuroghlian et al. 2015; Lee et al. 2015; Pennay et al. 2011.

[c]PTSD may be primary or secondary, depending on severity and on patient characteristics. See text for details.

Source. Adapted from Gunderson and Links 2014, p. 53.

tingencies for behavior management. Sobriety should also be incorporated into the crisis plan, including psychoeducation regarding triggers for use.

Common Problems

Patient Is Agitated or Potentially Suicidal

When patients are in severe distress, especially if they are suicidal, medication can reasonably be considered. No research has been done to date that clearly demonstrates whether medication is effective in such situations, but if nothing else, prescribing may generate a positive placebo effect. When faced with pressing requests to prescribe, clinicians who are skeptical of the utility of medication can negotiate and compromise, for example, offering 2 or 3 days of medication followed by reassessment. If there is a treatment team, be in contact with them before prescribing because the team may be able to brainstorm alternatives to medication. When adolescents report suicidal ideation, parents often need guidance as well. Explain the emergency precautions local to your area (e.g., paramedics, psychiatric response team, crisis hotline). In addition, discourage parents from making themselves responsible for keeping their child alive at home day and night. Adolescents in that degree of distress should be evaluated emergently to access a higher level of care.

Patient Is Nonadherent

Nonadherence is prevalent in health care generally; providers should make a point of inquiring about it. Common reasons for nonadherence include lack of perceived benefit, adverse effects, or failure to use reminders. Alternatively, family roles, communication, and independence may need to be addressed to establish whether adolescents or parents are tasked with taking or giving medication. Families may not realize or understand what is appropriate for a given adolescent's developmental level or may need guidance in negotiating a shared or graduated responsibility.

Patient Resists Medication Discontinuation

Overall, we recommend that medication(s) be discontinued over the medium term (months) unless they provide manifest benefit or if the entire family system strongly desires continuation. If initiating medication during a crisis, plan ahead to taper and discontinue after 1–3 weeks. This is especially true for antipsychotics. Ideally, discontinuation should take place on the basis of predetermined milestones (Simonsen et al. 2019). Milestones may include a lack of suicidal ideation or a functional improvement. When medications are long-standing, patients often avoid stopping them for fear of decompensation. However, it may be impossible to know or demonstrate the benefit of the medications without reducing the dose. Attempts to taper them can be suggested every 6–12 months.

Once a medication is started, patients or parents may express reluctance or outright refusal to stop it. Parents or patients often understandably fear a decompensation, and providers may even share these fears. Discuss fears openly, balanced against research showing limited effectiveness, against the limitations of existing research and against the patient's own behavior with the medication compared to without. In many instances patients are highly impaired despite (and perhaps because of) significant polypharmacy, calling into question the medication's effectiveness. Tracking mood and behavior (before, during, and after discontinuation) may lessen reluctance. Remind patients that changes can be reversed if previously uncertain benefits are revealed. At the same time, families need to expect spikes in emotion or maladaptive behavior when tapering or discontinuing an adolescent's medication. Such a deterioration could be consistent with the loss of a truly beneficial medication or with a negative placebo effect, coincidence, or unrelated life events. Nevertheless, be willing to continue medication if patients or parents insist, unless, of course side effects (e.g., rapid weight gain) pose a clear danger.

Patient Declines Medication

BPD symptoms can improve with or without medication, so it may be appropriate for a patient to decline pharmacotherapy. Listen to the reasons for declining to promote rapport. Give permission for patients to remain skeptical and ask them to share future concerns. Remind them that reliance on medication will be brief. Be willing to negotiate an alternative intervention, for example, completing a chain analysis of a behavior that would have been targeted with medication.

Divorced Parents Disagree With Each Other

It is problematic when both parents have legal custody and disagree about the use of medication. Ideally, hear out each parent and seek consensus.

Alternatively, a prescriber may negotiate with whichever parent opposes a recommended medication. The prescriber may offer to use a lower dose, treat for a shorter duration, or delay a defined amount of time before starting. Tracking a patient's mood and behavior—a good idea anyway—may also ameliorate a parent's suspicion about severity of illness or benefit of medication. In some instances, one parent opposes treatment and is otherwise unwilling to communicate with the provider. In those cases, the recourse is to the courts, or steps in that direction (e.g., letter from an attorney describing justification for proposed treatment), with a goal of motivating the parent to reconsider his or her position.

Patient Goes to College Outside the Local Area

The transition to college is a challenging one. There are inherent obstacles to the continuity and effectiveness of treatment, especially if the school is outside the clinician's local area. Patients face a major transition with academic and interpersonal stress, as well as greater temptation to use alcohol or drugs. In addition, new logistical barriers arise: college students move back and forth between cities and have irregular schedules. Given these difficulties, and in light of clinicians' increasing use of and comfort with telehealth, offering treatment virtually, as opposed to referring to a local provider, may enhance adherence to therapy and hence the effectiveness of treatment. This assertion is supported, albeit indirectly, by findings that telehealth as a modality is comparable (noninferior) to face-to-face treatment for insomnia or anxiety (American Academy of Child and Adolescent Psychiatry [AACAP] Committee on Telepsychiatry and AACAP Committee on Quality Issues 2017; Myers et al. 2017). Additional factors favoring telehealth include a lack of local referrals, low suicide risk or overall clinical severity, being in the middle or ending phase of treatment, and demonstrable progress in therapy. These considerations can be evaluated in cost-benefit decision-making and should allow the telehealth provider to be in contact with university health or residential services as needed in a way that is agreed on with the patient ahead of time.

Patient Has Been Diagnosed With Bipolar Disorder and Treated With Mood Stabilizers

BPD is often misdiagnosed as bipolar disorder (Bayes and Parker 2020). The implications of this for pharmacotherapy are significant. In bipolar disorder, medication is clearly indicated and will likely be a long-term intervention. Patients with BPD, on the other hand, may not even benefit from medication; it should be used briefly, if at all.

When adolescents present with a preexisting diagnosis of bipolar disorder, or a self-diagnosis, take a detailed history of any potential mania or hypomania. This will generally clarify whether bipolar disorder is absent or comorbid. In adults with BPD, a minority have co-occurring bipolar disorder that should be managed with indicated pharmacological interventions. Some patients identify strongly with the bipolar diagnosis, and you need not voice disagreement with that. Rather, psychoeducation is worthwhile. Mood lability in people with BPD is sometimes misunderstood, for example, as diagnostic of rapid-cycling bipolar disorder. Unfortunately, the term *rapid-cycling* is misleading. Although it would seem to suggest moods that change many times per day, in fact it refers to a form of bipolar disorder in which four or more episodes (cycles) of depression and hypomania occur in a *year*. Thus, even in rapid-cycling bipolar disorder, moods are episodic, not labile as in BPD.

If the patient is taking medication that you view as potentially unnecessary, encourage discontinuation using a rationale that the medication has not prevented the patient from seeking your services. Some patients may at least be willing to switch to a class of medication you recommend.

Chapter 7

Multimodal Treatments

Sara Rose Masland, Ph.D.
Carl Fleisher, M.D.

Rationale

It takes a village to raise a child. Adolescents grow up in a number of communities: at home, in school, and at extracurricular activities and work. Multimodal, or *split*, treatments are therefore common. Building your own support network in joining forces with another treater or modality can stabilize the treatment with a proper framework, particularly when the needs of patients with borderline personality disorder (BPD) and their families may exceed the capacity of a single clinician. When managed well, multimodal treatments can foster compliance with medications, reduce treatment-interfering behaviors, and decrease dropout for patients. They can also reduce burnout for clinicians.

Selecting Another Modality

The most common split-treatment structure includes a medical or psychiatric professional (psychiatrist, primary care pediatrician, or nurse practitioner) and an individual psychotherapist. Various treatment modalities and their complementary functions are listed in Table 7–1. When roles are clearly defined and communication is open, this arrangement generally works well. The good psychiatric management (GPM) mantra emphasizes work and doing one's job as well as clear delineation of roles that structure interactions. This applies to the interactions between treatment team members just as much as it applies to patients and their caregivers.

Family involvement is integral to the treatment. If family involvement is managed by a separate therapist, we generally recommend that a psychiatrist assume the role of individual therapy and medication management, a structure common in GPM for adults with BPD. However, in the context of adolescent treatment, some psychiatrists may feel more comfortable offering family guidance than individual therapy. A treatment structure in which the psychiatrist is responsible for medication management and family guidance may work well, particularly when the adolescent already has an individual therapist. Do not assume that patients require a psychotherapist *and* a separate family therapist—including either should follow needs rather than reflex.

A three-way split may also result from the involvement of a school-based treater. The degree of involvement from school counselors is likely to vary significantly. Some will have regular contact with adolescents and provide psychotherapy, whereas others may be more peripherally involved or may focus predominantly on academic testing and accommodations. When school counselors are involved, it is important to regard them as an integrated part of the treatment structure. Moreover, the school counselor is uniquely positioned to provide case management in the context of the adolescent's main "job": academics.

Although they are complex, three-way splits can work well if each clinician has a well-defined role. For example, clinicians should agree who will take the role of primary therapist—this person typically manages safety, evaluates progress, and leads treatment decisions (e.g., session frequency, referrals, how comorbidities will be handled, treatment termination). Clinicians should also agree on who will discuss and prescribe medications and how phone calls and inquiries from families will be han-

TABLE 7-1. Complementary treatment functions

Treatment modality	Function
Individual psychotherapy	Improve ability to think about one's own mental states and the mental states of others, explore issues of self, and identify and change cognitive and behavioral patterns.
Case management	Provide support for daily life, including for patients and their families. Insofar as parents handle planning, scheduling, transportation, and so on, they can be allies in case management.
School treatment	May serve a variety of functions (e.g., testing, accommodations, counseling). Treatment in school is most complementary when case management is provided.
Medication management	Medication, when used judiciously, may help with comorbid conditions.
Group therapy and/or group activities	Provide social support, social skills, coping skills, and identity development.
Family interventions	Provide support, decrease stress, promote functional communication.

Source. Adapted from Gunderson and Links 2014, p. 59.

dled. Providers should collaborate with one another, avoid vilification or marginalization of other treaters, and encourage the patient and family to voice any complaints directly to the appropriate treater.

Groups—therapeutic or extracurricular—provide a setting for socialization because they require consideration of others and one's impact on them. Socialization is essential for adolescent development and is also therapeutic for patients with BPD because it counterbalances the tendency to gravitate to exclusive relationships. Groups also provide an opportunity for adolescents to build supportive relationships with other adults, which may lessen the tendency to become dependent on the primary treater.

Common Problems With Setting the Treatment Frame

Many of the problems encountered when navigating multimodal treatments for adolescents occur when the treatment frame is questioned.

The Other Treater Resists the BPD Diagnosis

The problem of diagnostic resistance is a recurrent theme in the treatment of adolescents with BPD (see Chapter 3, "Making the Diagnosis and Providing Psychoeducation"). Making the diagnosis is critical to the GPM for adolescents (GPM-A) model because it sets the treatment frame and provides a shared understanding of the patient's difficulties. When another treater questions the diagnosis, this can threaten collaboration and erode trust in you. Use psychoeducation. The other treater may be open to your suggestions or at least to a compromise: they might agree that BPD is *likely* if the patient's current problems persist, and BPD should therefore be the target of intervention. When the other treater is noncommunicative or unconvinced, reevaluate the treatment structure.

The Other Treater Is Not Adhering to the Frame

Co-treaters may disrupt the GPM-A frame by suggesting or providing ineffective interventions. When communication and psychoeducation efforts have failed to forge an alliance between you and your co-treater, it may be time to discuss the treatment structure with your patient and their caregivers. Just as in family dynamics, it will be damaging for your adolescent patient to become the center of a dysfunctional dispute between two important adults, and provider changes should be made proactively.

The Other Treater Is Noncommunicative

Communication with other treaters, particularly prescribers, is essential yet often difficult to achieve regularly. Lack of communication may be acceptable, so long as the other treater is holding the frame and seeking feedback from you as appropriate. When the other treater makes interventions incompatible with your treatment plan and your communication efforts yield no response, enlist the parents, who can encourage the other provider to close the communication loop. If this fails, and there is evidence of harm or inappropriate prescribing, notify the other treater that you will recommend to your patient and the family that they consider changing providers. If the family insists on working with an uncollaborative treater, you may need to terminate care. Otherwise, you could end up complicit in a treatment more likely to cause harm than to help.

Parents Have Difficulty Holding the Frame

Parents are potent allies in navigating the complexities of a split treatment. However, they may also have difficulty holding the frame. They may wish for one treater to have a more central role than another or may, at times, disagree with treatment goals and interventions. This is likely when one or both parents feel a stronger connection with one treater than the other, when one treater marginalizes the efforts of another, or when parents have divergent views on which treaters (and modalities) are most important. It is important to provide psychoeducation about treatments and the potential for a multimodal treatment to create harmful splits between family members and treaters. You should actively seek collaboration with parents to ensure that all parties communicate and work toward shared goals.

Groups: Therapy and Extracurriculars

The benefit of group therapy is less clear for adolescents with BPD than for adults. Group therapy approaches found effective for adult patients with BPD have not yet shown consistent effectiveness for adolescents in treatment trials (Beck et al. 2016; Schuppert et al. 2009, 2012). Instead, recent developments suggest that a focus on the social context in which the adolescent normally operates (e.g., school, extracurricular activities, clubs) may be more useful (see Bo et al. 2017; Fonagy and Allison 2014; Luyten et al. 2020).

Until more evidence supports group therapy for adolescents with BPD, GPM-A encourages a focus on involvement in extracurricular activities as an alternative. Although adolescents with BPD participate in extracurricular groups less often than do those without BPD (Kramer et al. 2017b), these groups have shown significant benefits for teens in fostering formation of new friendships, greater well-being, better health, lower depressive symptoms, less disruptive behavior, and more positive attitudes toward school (Darling 2005; Driessens 2015; Mason et al. 2009; Oberle et al. 2019; Schaefer et al. 2011). One of the main benefits of groups is the opportunity for social learning. Participation in activities such as clubs (e.g., 4-H, math team, drama club, band, chorus) or team sports may be further conducive to identity formation and goal pursuit. Teenagers are usually busy finding out what they like and what they are good at, which increases motivation and self-esteem. Adolescents should be required to participate in some kind of group—extracurriculars should receive first priority, but group therapy is still also an option. Group therapy may be a stepping stone when the adolescent is too overwhelmed to get involved in a community-based extracurricular activity.

Resistance to engaging in extracurriculars and group therapy is likely to depend on the adolescent's interpersonal hypersensitivity and experience with peer group rejection. Provide psychoeducation to adolescents and parents about the value of group involvement. Groups—extracurricular or therapeutic—provide tools for developing new coping strategies, offer valuable perspectives on how patients may be acting in ways that harm relationships, and provide feedback on how to change problematic behaviors.

Therapeutic groups provide a safe space in which adolescents can learn to share their own difficulties—thereby reducing feelings of shame and isolation—while learning to make space for others. When other people speak, adolescents have the opportunity to observe them express and explore feelings that they themselves may typically avoid. As an added benefit, when adolescents come to know peers with similar problems, this can help them accept the reality of their own situation. Learning to navigate participation in a group, including self-other awareness, and the need to make space for others fosters the development of important social skills, including empathic listening, sharing, engaging with others noncompetitively, and relating to others nonromantically.

A number of specific or specialized group treatments, as well as self-help or specialized support groups (e.g., Alcoholics Anonymous) may be useful for adolescents with BPD, but these are often expensive or unavailable, especially for adolescents. Secondary schools and colleges sometimes offer groups on campus, and more mature adolescents may be able to use adult-focused groups. Skills groups in particular complement GPM-A well when approached as a means to learn interpersonal and functional skills to cope with interpersonal hypersensitivity and emotional reactivity. The didactic and structured nature of these groups will be familiar to school-age adolescents and may therefore induce less stress than do process-oriented groups. Regardless of the group's particular orientation, good communication between the primary clinician and group treater will facilitate the group's helpfulness (see earlier subsection "The Other Treater is Noncommunicative").

Common Problems in Group Therapy

Interfering Behaviors

It is not uncommon for an adolescent patient to willfully disengage from group therapy or actively deride the treatment or group leader. Before group therapy begins, the primary treater should outline expectations for the group process. It is also useful to make the prediction that group will be challenging at times and the adolescent may feel pulled to disrupt or disengage. Group leaders should respond actively to behaviors that interfere with the group process, ideally during the group. Alternatively, rather than call a disruptive patient *out*, a group leader can call the patient *in*, relying on group process and the spirit of collaboration. Group leaders must use their best judgment in so doing because there is the potential for this strategy to lead to further distraction.

> It seems like you are having some difficulty engaging with the group, and it has become hard for us to stay on track. I'm concerned, and I wonder if there is some way that we, as a group, can support your engagement today? Is there a skill you have learned that may be useful to practice right now?

When this kind of gentle redirecting, with expression of concern and care, is not effective, or when it leads to further behaviors that derail the group's agenda, direct conversations with patients, and potentially families, can occur between sessions. If adolescents do not respond to repeated active efforts to engage them productively, they should be suspended from group with the option to continue "when ready." Suspension from group therapy should not affect involvement in group extracurriculars but rather suggests that an adolescent may benefit more from extracurricular involvement than from a therapeutic group.

> I've noticed that you are having difficulty engaging in the group effectively. As we have discussed before, it is very important that everyone in the group work together—this is a team—and there continue to be times when you do things that take the group off track. [Provide patient-specific examples here, as needed.]
>
> I recognize that it can sometimes be very difficult to engage effectively with your peers, and this may not be the right time for you to continue with group treatment. At this time, I think it makes sense for you to take a break from the group. You will be very welcome to join the group again when you are ready to engage effectively. [Provide patient-specific examples of what "readiness" looks like.] I still believe that this group can be very helpful to you, and I hope that you are able to join again in the future.

Behavioral Contagion

Group treatments that focus on emotion regulation may have particular importance in reducing nonsuicidal self-injury (NSSI).[1] However, groups also pose some risks for the initiation or maintenance of NSSI. Notably, lack of awareness about NSSI is a significant barrier to engaging in NSSI (Hooley and Franklin 2018), adolescents may reinforce one another's NSSI behaviors (Granic and Dishion 2003), and some adolescents gain peer group affiliation

---

[1]Therapy groups are not the only source of behavioral contagion. Adolescents are exposed to NSSI through their peers and the media. Of particular note, online groups and communities are increasingly popular sources of information and support. Adolescents are using Twitter, Reddit, and similar online communities in greater numbers (although Facebook use among adolescents is declining in favor of these other platforms). Much of what adolescents are exposed to on these platforms is useful. However, these communities sometimes go so far as to explicitly condone or support the use of NSSI (and other behaviors, including disordered eating). Talk with your adolescent patients about their use of these communities and be prepared to offer alternative sources of self-help or online support.

or a boost in self-image by adopting peers' NSSI behaviors (Cohen and Prinstein 2006; Giletta et al. 2013; Hooley and Franklin 2018; Prinstein et al. 2010). NSSI is often used when adolescents have difficulty with emotion regulation (e.g., Fox et al. 2015; Franklin et al. 2010; Hasking et al. 2017; Nock et al. 2009; Robinson et al. 2019). Before group treatment begins, provide psychoeducation about the reasons people self-harm and the reasons they should not and discuss adaptive strategies for emotion regulation and peer affiliation. To the extent possible, match patients to groups with narrow age ranges (e.g., 12–14 years, 15–17 years). This will avoid situations in which younger adolescents are unduly influenced by reports of NSSI or other self-harming or impulsive behavior by older adolescents.

Interpersonal Issues With Group Members

Adolescents are particularly sensitive to the approval of social groups. In a group setting—therapeutic or extracurricular—they may form exclusive relationships with peers, including enmeshed and exclusionary dyads or, less commonly, larger cliques. Forming relationships with other group members may be useful, so long as it does not interfere with treatment. This is an opportunity for psychoeducation about 1) the tendency for people with BPD to form exclusive relationships that ultimately perpetuate interpersonal dysfunction and 2) the importance of placing work (in this case, the work of therapy, academics, and engagement with valued activities) before love (both romantic and platonic in this context).

> For people with BPD, there is a tendency to form very intense one-on-one relationships with others, romantic or just between friends. Although it is natural to desire a "best friend," exclusive and intense relationships can cause problems over time. For example, when something happens in the relationship—perhaps you feel rejected, have an argument, or the other person finds a new close friend or moves away—this can be extremely dysregulating, particularly when you have really come to depend on that person. Because we will all be getting to know one another in this group, you may find yourself starting to form these kinds of relationships with one another. I want us to collaboratively keep an eye on that and to avoid it whenever possible.

If adolescents ask you what signs might indicate they are forming an intense kind of exclusive relationship with someone, you can first ask them what they think, then add the following:

> Some other signs include that you are hanging out or talking to only one other group member. You might be in contact with that person very frequently and are relying on them to help you when you are struggling instead of relying on the things you learn in this group or individual therapy. You are jealous or feel rejected when that person talks with other friends or group members, or you are purposely excluding or gossiping about other group members. And during this group, one guideline we will follow is that there should not be any romantic relationships between group members. We know that adolescents with BPD symptoms are more involved in romantic relationships than those without BPD, and that relationship intensity makes it more likely for BPD symptoms to continue. I want you to feel comfortable speaking in group and to get to know one another, but let's make sure that we use this as a chance to build healthy relationships.

Group leaders can also explain why it would be wise to stay aware of the intensity or exclusivity of one's relationships.

> In this group, we also want you to find ways to build a life of purpose and meaning that does not depend on intense or exclusive relationships. When you find ways to engage with school and extracurricular groups, this has a stabilizing effect. Building a life that does not depend on intense attachment to others will help you find a sense of identity, regulate your emotions, and be resilient in the face of challenges. It will also give you opportunities to practice building strong, healthy, nonexclusive relationships with your peers. For these reasons, one philosophy of this group will be "school before love" or "life before love."

Parents should receive this psychoeducation as well because they may provide transportation and supervision for intersession relationships. Intersession friendships often seem benign and even beneficial at first but evolve into problems over time. When these intersession relationships interfere with group process or participation or perpetuate impulsive or self-damaging behavior, this should be addressed within the group, and primary clinicians can evaluate the group's helpfulness.

Absences

Consistent attendance is important, both to ensure that the individual patient benefits from the group and to nurture group process. Discuss repeated absences with the patient and their parents, and enlist parents to be firm about attendance. If absences are consistent, terminate treatment with the option to resume in the future.

Family Interventions

Caregiver involvement typically is essential for adolescent treatment because it allows clinicians to assess family strengths and dysfunctions and support family members who bear a heavy burden in trying to negotiate challenging behaviors (see Chapter 4, "Getting Started," and Appendix D, "Guidelines for Families"). That said, this need not take the form of full family therapy. Table 7–2 describes family interventions and selection guidelines. Family therapy is the least common type of family intervention, reserved for those families for whom communication and collaboration are strong enough to support the exploration of systems problems. When a separate family therapist is not involved, one treater should be designated to meet with parents on a regular or semiregular basis to provide psychoeducation and support and to foster a strong alliance, which is critical to keeping the adolescent engaged in treatment.

Discussing the Role of Parents and Confidentiality With the Patient

Adolescent patients have realistic concerns about how much of your discussion will be shared with their parents or guardians. These concerns, and the limits of confidentiality, should be among the first topics of discussion. Specifically, patients should know that their parents will be informed about safety issues, threats to life, and the structure and expectations of treatment but will not receive detailed information about what happens in each session. It is best to approach issues of confidentiality with a collaborative tone—avoidance of an authoritarian tone will help set the frame of mutual respect. Adolescents should be aware of family therapist communications. Adolescents may also have concerns about the degree to which their parents are involved in treatment more generally. You can assure them that one goal of treatment is to help their parents (and other family members) better understand them and enable their independence.

Enlisting Parental Participation and Delineating Boundaries

The pull for intrusive overinvolvement or, conversely, helpless disengagement, may be strong for parents who are frightened by impulsive or self-harming behaviors. Parents will need to both trust you as an expert and understand your limitations as a human. It is important to set the frame

TABLE 7–2. Hierarchy of family interventions for adolescents with borderline personality disorder (BPD)

Type of intervention	Features	Comments
Psychoeducation	Information about the disorder (diagnosis, causes, prognosis) should be provided to all family members. The content and complexity may need to be scaled for the patient's younger siblings. Psychoeducation should also include information about parenting a child with BPD.	For family guidelines, see Appendix D.
Counseling (up to and including individual therapy for family members)	Family guidelines should be provided in counseling sessions with parents and/or family. You may handle some additional counseling sessions, particularly for parents seeking further guidance or general advice.	Counseling is intended for parents and other family members, including siblings. When additional counseling or individual therapy is indicated for parents or siblings, make a referral. Their individual treatment should be considered separate from the treatment of your patient.
Support groups	Support groups (e.g., Family Connections[a]) might focus on the family or parenting.	General parenting support groups may be useful in the absence of BPD-specific groups. Clinics should develop support groups as needed.

TABLE 7–2.   **Hierarchy of family interventions for adolescents with borderline personality disorder (BPD)** *(continued)*

Type of intervention	Features	Comments
Conjoint sessions (patients and caregivers)	Conjoint sessions are useful for setting the treatment frame and reviewing the importance of collaboration, limits of confidentiality, and the importance (and limits of) the patient's independence or agency. You can help broker problem-solving and assist in planning (e.g., budgets, schedules, sleep hygiene, access to vehicles, time away with and without the adolescent, handling emergencies).	These sessions can quickly broker agreements that are essential to case management, which provides structure and predictability for patients and their family.
Couples therapy	Primary clinicians should lead couples sessions as needed. If parental discord is significant and frequent sessions are needed or parental conflict occupies much of the treatment focus, separate couples work is recommended.	Couples therapy is useful for enlisting collaboration, decreasing splitting, and reducing stress in the patient's home environment.
Mediation	Estranged parents may need outside legal counsel to establish co-parenting guidelines.	Mediation structures co-parent communication on a legal basis when it is otherwise difficult to broker constructive engagement.

TABLE 7–2. Hierarchy of family interventions for adolescents with borderline personality disorder (BPD) *(continued)*

Type of intervention	Features	Comments
Family therapy	Family therapy may be used to improve communication patterns and target specific sources of family dysfunction.	Family therapy is contraindicated for families who cannot discuss conflict without escalation.

[a]Sponsored by National Education Alliance for Borderline Personality Disorder/National Alliance on Mental Illness.

Source. Adapted from Gunderson and Links 2014, p. 64.

for involvement early in treatment: parents are essential for reinforcing treatment interventions at home but must also work to foster their child's independence, even in the context of challenging behaviors. When two or more parents are involved, they may often disagree with one another about treatment approaches and targets. Conjoint sessions will be important for enlisting unified support and also for identifying cases that require marital counseling or mediation.

Alliance Building

As with adult patients, the treatment alliance may be reliably established with support, psychoeducation, and collaboration.

Support

Caregivers are likely to feel (but not necessarily express) a range of emotions, including hopelessness, fear, and shame. They may be experiencing significant emotional and/or financial distress. Your first step should be to encourage them to discuss their experience and to validate and recognize the difficulties they have encountered. Support will naturally turn to psychoeducation as you assure them that their efforts have failed not because they did not do all that they could but because their child has special needs that require responses that do not come naturally to most parents. These responses may be quite different from what helped them ensure that their other children could flourish.

Psychoeducation

Psychoeducation should be an early and recurrent aspect of treatment and provides a foundation for giving feedback on parenting skills or the need for parenting support groups. The first phase of psychoeducation, which should be offered to all parents and their spouses, focuses on the disorder itself and is critical for setting expectations and dispelling common myths or sources of shame for families.

Parents will usually want to know what causes BPD. The framework of interactions between genetics (or biology more broadly) and environment is useful.

> The causes of BPD are complex and involve the interaction of predispositions and the environment. Predispositions are things you may have noticed in your child even as an infant. These can include significant negative emotionality (intense moods) or interpersonal sensitivity (depending too much on relationships). These are often present even from birth because they are inherited. BPD is significantly heritable—more so than depression and anxiety disorders. There is no single gene that causes BPD, and it depends on the interaction of many different genes, as well as the interaction of those genes with the environment.

Parents who read about their adolescent's diagnosis may grow concerned about the research on childhood trauma as a causal factor of BPD.

> Indeed, the majority of patients with BPD do report neglect and either physical or sexual abuse. Although these are common, they are not required for BPD to develop, nor are they sufficient in and of themselves. Many children with BPD have not had these experiences, and many children have these experiences but do not develop BPD.

Clinicians can also educate parents on other early environmental factors that contribute to BPD. Parents and children affect one another reciprocally (Stepp et al. 2014b), and it is natural for parents to wonder what happened and if they are at fault. Psychoeducation can help mitigate feelings of blame.

> Children can be born with excessive negative emotionality or interpersonal hypersensitivity, which means that they have different needs than other children and are more difficult to parent. Meeting these needs may not come easily to you, especially if you are stressed or anxious yourself, or if you have other children who also need attention. It is hard to be continually calm or involved in order to soothe a reactive infant.

Parents may also have significant fears about the long-term functioning of their child. Although the future is uncertain, you can rely on studies of the longitudinal course of BPD to provide a hopeful message.

> Although you may sometimes feel hopeless, it is important to remember that BPD is an illness that responds to treatment and also naturally improves over time. This treatment is meant to accelerate the natural process of recovery, and although your child may always need additional supports for optimal functioning, you can expect that their frightening behaviors, impulsivity, and aggression will diminish over time.

It is also useful to present the interpersonal hypersensitivity model very early in the treatment (for guidance, see Figure 2–1 in Chapter 2, "Overall Principles," and Chapter 3, "Making the Diagnosis and Providing Psychoeducation"). Parents are likely to see the cycle of connectedness, threatened hostility, alienated aloneness, and despairing suicidality play out at home or may be able to reflect on how the cycle has led them to the current treatment. They should be enlisted to observe patterns consistent with the model and to help their child do the same.

Collaboration

Encourage parents to collaborate actively. Articulate a clear role for them, in which they are there to support the treatment and their child. They can support treatment by addressing you directly when they have concerns or questions and encouraging communication between treatment providers. They can support their child by recognizing the limitations that accompany interpersonal hypersensitivity and difficulties with self-control and by working to take a nonreactive stance.

Siblings

When the patient has siblings, you should also consider their needs for support and make recommendations. Parents often welcome referrals for their other children. At other times, however, they may hesitate because they may have limited resources, have difficulty confronting the idea that their other children have been affected, or see their other children's problems as minor in comparison to the struggles of their child with BPD. It will be important to emphasize that siblings of adolescents with BPD often express distress about their sibling's difficulties and the family impacts of those difficulties (e.g., Giffin 2008). Although many siblings of children with BPD show significant resilience (e.g., Laporte et al. 2011; Paris et al. 2014), family members of adolescents with BPD are more likely than the general population to experience psychopathology, including anxiety and mood disorders (Bandelow et al. 2005) and ADHD (Kuja-Halkola et al. 2018). Siblings can benefit from therapeutic support even when they are not outwardly expressing difficulties—*they often struggle silently.* Providing them with support outside the family can alleviate parent burden. Trusted adult social support outside the family may also buffer against the development of BPD in siblings (Paris et al. 2014).

Parent and family psychoeducation is likely to be helpful to both patients and their siblings. The family dynamics among adolescents with BPD are often characterized by significant conflict, including criticism, emotional overinvolvement (Bailey and Grenyer 2015), anger, and irritability (James and Vereker 1996). These aspects of the family environment are often reciprocally reinforced among patients and caregivers (Fruzzetti et al. 2005; Hahlweg et al. 1989; Hooley 1990; Simoneau et al. 1998). Families who express higher levels of criticism do not typically do so malevolently—they are often motivated by a desire to help the patient and the belief that the patient can do more to change (see Hooley 2007). Psychoeducation reduces these patterns of expressed emotion and conflict for other illnesses (e.g., Eisler et al. 2000; Fristad et al. 1998; Honig et al. 1997; Kim and Miklowitz 2004) and is likely to do the same for BPD, with broad benefits for the family system.

Common Problems in Family Interventions

Patient or Parents Demand Changes to Confidentiality

Parents or the patient predictably question or test the limits of confidentiality. In the wake of alarming impulsivity or self-harming behaviors, parents may feel a sense of powerlessness that drives them to seek answers and assert greater control. They may insist that you provide more details about your sessions with their child. In this situation, you can fall back on the principles of support and collaboration. Validate their concerns and express that you understand why they would like more information. Parents also need to know that their extreme reactions may actually reinforce these kinds of behaviors. You can offer reassurance that you will provide detailed information when it is necessary to keep their child safe. Enlist them to collaborate with you to ensure that the treatment is successful, which necessarily relies on their child trusting you to respect their confidentiality as agreed.

Your adolescent patients also may seek to renegotiate rules around confidentiality when they wish to disclose information to you that would upset their parents (e.g., drug use, sexual behaviors, questions about identity, self-harm, rule violations). When patients disclose information to you that you feel should be relayed to their parents, this is an opportunity to facilitate their own agency. Provide them guidance in negotiating the disclosure with their parents. This will position the disclosure of information as an opportunity for growth and self-controlled communication rather than a breach of trust.

When parents are estranged or family dynamics are contentious, parents may ask you for session information that supports their position or potential litigation. In other cases, they may wish for you to communicate information about their child to outside clinicians or parties (e.g., schools, lawyers) in ways that have not been agreed on previously. When confidentiality is tested or questioned or when a disclosure is necessary, it can be useful to have a conjoint session in which parents and adolescents can express their concerns. Offer conjoint sessions only if you believe that the family can engage productively.

A Parent or Adolescent Makes Allegations of Abuse

The majority of adults with BPD report childhood abuse or neglect. Parents, particularly those who are estranged, may also make allegations of abuse against one another. When working with adolescents, you have a responsibility to act as a mandated reporter when you have reasonable suspicion of current or ongoing abuse.

Inquire about abuse or neglect in a one-on-one conversation with the adolescent during your assessment. Remind patients that talking to you is confidential and explain that part of your job is to make sure no one hurts them or treats them inappropriately. You may start with general questions: "Do you feel safe at home?" "What happens when people get angry at you?" "Is there a particular person you fear?" Alternatively, be direct and ask if anyone has hit or hurt them or whether they have been touched, or been told to touch someone else, inappropriately.

If an adolescent has experienced abuse or neglect, it is meaningful to say first that such behavior is wrong and that no one deserves to be treated that way by anyone. If the abuse or neglect is current (or recent), you must then ask about the circumstances and establish your own judgment as to whether it is safe for the adolescent to return home from your office. In the case of physical or sexual abuse, for example, it may be necessary to make an emergency report with child protective services, who can find the adolescent a safe place to stay that same day. In less severe cases, or with uncertain or intermittent incidents, you may decide against making a report immediately but instead ask more questions about extent, duration, frequency, location, tangible injury, triggers, and sibling involvement.

It is helpful to understand how child protective services investigates a claim and the resources available to that local agency. For example, although most agencies are limited to protective or punitive measures for documented abuse, some agencies can offer families educational or therapeutic resources. Moreover, not all abuse can be acted on readily: emotional abuse is one of the most common forms of maltreatment yet is difficult to prove.

The decision to report may be influenced by your understanding of what will come of such an action, balancing the potential benefits and risks. Risks to be mindful of include 1) being perceived as vilifying the parents, 2) creating or perpetuating a victim identity for your patient, and 3) damaging the patient's trust by disclosing information that was shared in confidence. Any of these risks, particularly the first and third outcomes, may lead to further harm in the form of termination of treatment even when the situation is handled impeccably. In some instances, providers may need to consider whether an adolescent is better served by remaining in effective treatment versus no treatment plus what—if anything—comes of an investigation by child protective services.

You may decide to monitor the situation rather than report a vague suspicion immediately. In the case of neglect or emotional abuse by parents, delaying reporting can clarify the best course of action by creating an opportunity to evaluate the effectiveness of your treatment in terms of improving the family's interactions.

When a report is appropriate, you should educate the patient and family about what to expect. Give as much information as possible, including actions ("Someone will call or come to the house"), timing ("tomorrow" or "within a week"), who will be involved ("a caseworker from the state/county"), process ("After they interview everyone, they will make a determination and file a report"), and outcome ("They may suggest helpful resources, require you to take a class, or refer the matter to the police"). When possible, you should frame your report as a supportive, collaborative intervention that views parents as having good intentions. For example, you may highlight that parents can feel overwhelmed with such an emotional child and/or normalize that any parent would welcome support and suggestions in dealing with challenging situations.

Parents Are Noncollaborative or Disengaged

An engaged parent is not necessarily a helpful parent, and it is critical that parents understand and agree with the need for collaboration. Provide psychoeducation and transparency around your clinical decision-making. This will help parents view you as an expert who cares about their participation. When parents actively deride the treatment with each other or to other people (e.g., other treaters, their child), address this early and directly. Assess where they disagree with your approach and explain the importance of maintaining the treatment frame consistently.

Fearfulness may be expressed in a number of ways (e.g., coddling, withdrawal, unrealistic demands, blaming self or others, litigiousness). It is important both to expect this in families of young people with BPD and to normalize it as a starting point. It is more likely that parents will be over-engaged in therapy in reaction to fear or misguided attempts to be helpful, but the opposite pattern is not uncommon. Some parents may be difficult to engage in therapy altogether. Similar guidelines apply to both scenarios: provide psychoeducation and transparency, actively enlist parents' support and understanding, assess points of disagreement and address them directly, and instruct parents on how to engage more constructively.

When these steps fail to enlist productive participation, document your recommendations. If you provide proper education and opportunity to be involved, you have implemented a standard of care, leaving the family to choose to follow recommendations or not. Consider termination as a last resort only if the interaction between the treatment and family proves to be unhelpful or harmful to the patient.

Estranged Parents or Stepparents Disagree About Their Roles

Family splits are a reality for many adolescents. Even parents who are not estranged may have significant disagreements about what is best for their child and may attempt to enlist your support for their views. This is true when working with any estranged parents and particularly common for parents of children with BPD. When it becomes difficult to avoid entanglement in parental disagreements, recommend couples therapy, mediation, or a parental support group. You should also be very clear with parents that it is important for the adolescent to have consistent rules, support, and expectations across households. Rules and expectations should be discussed explicitly, and parents should refrain from blaming each other for their child's difficulties.

Divorced parents may disagree about the extent to which stepparents should contribute to family decisions, including treatment planning. Use an "it takes a village" approach with families. Encourage the inclusion of stepparents in treatment planning, and even in conjoint sessions, when it serves to foster collaboration and support rather than escalate dysfunction or splitting. The extent to which this is possible depends on parental willingness, as well as the adolescent's acceptance. Help families to delineate clear roles for each caregiver and to determine how important decisions will be made.

School-Based Treatments
Middle and High School Services

During the academic year, adolescents spend the majority of their time at school. The challenges of academics, combined with the usually intense interpersonal negotiations of teenagers, create a situation in which difficulties are likely to manifest at school. However, because the school environment often has a great deal of structure, some adolescents may be more stable at school than at home. Regardless, school treaters and resources may be useful.

The "work" of adolescence includes academics and school-based extracurricular activities. School treaters (e.g., school psychologists, mental health counselors, general guidance counselors) can offer useful case management to support this work. It is important to communicate the GPM-A treatment frame to school treaters, to emphasize the benefits of structure, and to offer suggestions for academic accommodations that support the student without coddling or perpetuating avoidance. These accommodations should be specific and predictable rather than vague and reactive to emotional stress. To facilitate communication with school treaters, parents may need to sign releases and actively encourage communication.

College Mental Health Services

People with BPD are most likely to present to treatment for the first time at the transition to adulthood (Hersh 2013; Zanarini et al. 2001). This is also the time at which many adolescents will begin college, where the relative lack of structure, potential distance from home, introduction to new interpersonal situations, and access to substances present many challenges.

When a patient begins college, discuss whether treatment should continue. If the college is far from home and your location, a referral to a clinician who specializes in personality disorders may be appropriate. You may agree to see the patient when they are home during long breaks or to act as a consultant to treaters in the new location. If no suitable provider is available, you can consider telehealth sessions or work with the patient to identify other treatment resources, including the college or university mental health center. Most colleges and universities have mental health centers and may provide a range of group treatments, including support groups and skills groups. These are an excellent option for continued care.

Colleges and universities often offer support and mental health services outside the designated counseling center. For example, many have organizations designed to provide support to historically underrepresented students (e.g., an Office of Black Student Affairs), LGBTQ+ students, women, or survivors of sexual violence. These centers may run support and/or skills groups. Additionally, a college is likely to have administrators, some with counseling backgrounds, designated for student support in a Dean of Students office or similar organization. The degree to which individuals in these offices are willing to communicate with you may vary. However, if you continue to treat an adolescent through their college experience, it will be useful to view these services through the lens of a split treatment.

Common Problems With School Treatment

Concerns About Stigma

Families of people with BPD often face discrimination and stigma from health professionals (Lawn and McMahon 2015). Similarly, patients and parents may fear and experience stigmatization from school administrators. Unfortunately, this fear is appropriate in many cases and may create resistance to involving school treaters. Collaborate with patients and parents to determine whether the benefits of involving schools outweigh the potential risks and be willing to reach out to school treaters to facilitate as necessary. Sometimes, providers may minimize stigma by describing pertinent challenges to school treaters but withholding diagnostic information. That way, because the patient's symptoms may already be quite evident, school treaters can still facilitate appropriate coping strategies.

Lack of Treatment Access

In recent years, colleges across the United States have seen increasing demand for mental health services and are often spread thin (Benton et al. 2003; Kitzrow 2003). This creates access difficulties, including significant wait lists, caps on the number of sessions offered, and inflexibility about frequency of sessions. Adolescents with BPD may have difficulty accessing care while at college, which is particularly troubling if they are some distance from home. It is rare to find BPD-specific treatments at college mental health centers. Indeed, reluctance to diagnose BPD is common in these settings. When your patient is actively engaged in a college search, you can encourage them, perhaps in collaboration with a school counselor, to select a school with strong mental health services or in a location where you can make an appropriate referral. The National Alliance on Mental Illness provides guidelines for selecting colleges and universities with mental health services in mind (www.nami.org/Find-Support/Teens-Young-Adults/Managing-a-Mental-Health-Condition-in-College). If many of your patients attend a particular local university or college, organizing a GPM training for campus providers or referring them to online training resources (Appendix C, "Online Good Psychiatric Management Training") may be useful.

Hospitalizations

Hospitalizations are rarely helpful for adolescents with BPD, but college mental health clinicians and student support administrators may apply a cautious approach to treatment by making hospitalization or "transport" decisions that are not in the student's best interest. They are unlikely to be flexible in their approach, but communication of your concerns is still warranted. If you have a patient with a history of hospitalizations or who is likely to be hospitalized while away at college, identify a primary clinician with a personality disorders specialty in the patient's new location if possible. This provider may be better able to navigate the intricacies of the local hospital system.

Threats to the Treatment Frame

Secondary schools in the United States are highly structured. This structure supports the GPM treatment frame but may disappear altogether when a patient begins postsecondary education. In many college or university settings, students find themselves in class for as little as 10 hours per week. They must necessarily work to structure their time outside class—a significant challenge for adolescents with BPD. You should both prepare your patient for this abrupt shift and work with school providers to plan ahead. Many well-meaning administrators will quickly provide accommodations, including excused absences, excused tardiness, or alternative deadlines. These accommodations may be useful for many mental health conditions, and sometimes they are useful for students with BPD. However, they are more likely to erode necessary structure and undermine GPM's focus on work.

Chapter 8

Ending Treatment

Lois W. Choi-Kain, M.D., M.Ed., DFAPA
Carla Sharp, Ph.D.

ENDING TREATMENT TAKES MANY FORMS
with adolescent patients. Transitions, dropouts, and terminations bring
treatment to a pause or an ending in both expected and unexpected ways.
Adolescents in general are more difficult to engage in lengthy treatments
than are adults. When adolescents' attention turns to building relationships with peers and activities in their communities, caregivers should let
go and provide space for independence and growth. For this reason, many
of the evidence-based treatments for borderline personality disorder
(BPD) adapted to adolescents are brief by design (see Table A–1 in Appendix A, "Relation of Good Psychiatric Management for Adolescents to

Other Evidence-Based Treatments for Adolescent Borderline Personality Disorder"). We encourage offering good psychiatric management for adolescents (GPM-A) in a flexible format. You can start with a short-term commitment for a specific number of sessions (see Chapter 4, "Getting Started"). These short stretches allow the teen, the family, and you a chance to both collaborate on short-term goals and evaluate the treatment for its effectiveness in manageable chunks. Also, it gives pause for adolescents to figure out what they need, which will change as they make progress, and puts them in charge of asking for what they want in a way that is credible.

Shorter-term commitment to care also provides many opportunities for tapering frequency and ending in a planned way. For adolescents with BPD, saying goodbye allows exposure to the many mixed emotions about your relationship with them, as well as their work of managing without you, whether it means less frequent appointments or a more permanent termination. Whenever possible, offer booster sessions for times of high stress or important transitions. If compatible with your practice setting, allow follow-up the way a primary care provider would for an annual checkup. Being available in a predictable, albeit infrequent, way socializes the teen you treated for BPD for regular health maintenance rather than crisis-oriented care.

Whether termination is mutually agreed on or not, be clear about what you recommend, why, and how you can help the patient and his or her family evaluate the costs and benefits of continuing. If the patient drops out unexpectedly, provide an opportunity for another appointment to discuss his or her reasons in a time-limited window. Patients' reasons may vary, from a sense that they have gotten what they needed to being too troubled to engage in treatment (O'Keeffe et al. 2019). Sometimes you may recommend termination because the treatment is not effective. In these cases, you can be clear about what would be needed for treatment to be more effective and make referrals.

When termination is planned, few patients with BPD leave treatment with mourning, especially in adolescence. Most leave with anxieties that may be eased with reassurances of ongoing availability. Internalization of a soothing other is gradual, and the corrective experience of your relationship will be most meaningful if the teen builds some confidence to move forward without you. That is, after all, the adolescent's job. You can expect that abandonment fears will diminish before intolerance of aloneness. Review what the patient has learned to manage this vulnerability.

We offer a few general tips on termination. Termination itself should be time-limited and have an end point. Once you, the patient, and the family agree on termination, set aside a specific number of sessions for it. More sessions will be needed for planning transitions (e.g., relocations, departure for college), but the time you need to say goodbye can span one to three sessions. You can ask patients to write a short story or draw a cartoon about different moments in their treatment, from where they were when they started to where they finished. This prompts them to think autobiographically to provide a sense of coherence and identity. You can also ask them to think about the future, stressful situations they might encounter, and what they imagine you would say in those situations. In so doing, patients learn they know you well enough to conjure a sense of how you might guide them, even when you are not around. Encourage independent living skills as a preparation for young adulthood while also reminding patients how they will know they need help. Put as much as you can down on paper. The termination process, once started, is often emotional for teens, making it hard for them to process the toolkit that you are busy putting together for relapse prevention. Therefore, concrete notes about skills learned and solutions for expected challenges will facilitate retention. Involving family in this process is welcome. Their involvement at the ending can provide appreciation of gains made and direction for the future.

Termination will not always go smoothly. Teens with BPD will be sensitive to the separation, as will their parents. You can respond to expression of strong emotions, predicted by the interpersonal hypersensitivity model, as an opportunity to remind the patient and family what they have learned in your work together. Remind them of their vulnerabilities to interpersonal stress and ways they have managed it by thinking first, developing trusting relationships, and getting a life. Reflect on teens' progress in awareness of themselves and the way social interactions work. Point out ways they have learned to learn rather than remain rigid and stuck. Reorient them to getting a life by building social capital, engaging others through shared interests and activities, and building self-esteem. Counterbalance the confidence you express in their moves forward with appreciation of what it takes to do so.

Working with adolescents with BPD can be a highly rewarding experience. They will need your help and can get better. Some will remit, and others will continue to have some symptoms. Treatment can help without having to be a total cure. We hope this handbook provides enough advice to steady you in the process. In offering the GPM-A approach, you can be satisfied in addressing a public health problem in a cost-effective and available way. We hope the experience of working with adolescents with BPD generates pride in your skills. The capacities to manage the care of

BPD will have utility in the treatment of other patients and perhaps more broadly in your life. We have found that working with patients with BPD also fuels personal growth, aiding all of us to be less reactive (slowing down) and more thoughtful with experience. This work can prove deeply appreciated by patients, even when the treatment is not an immediate success, and has the potential to be life-changing.

In the original *Handbook of Good Psychiatric Management for Border-line Personality Disorder*, John Gunderson wrote:

> In retrospect, most of what I learned seems quite obvious. I hope that readers will find this true for them. I do not see myself as particularly gifted, and I do not believe that only experts can be effective treaters. I do believe that I have become "good enough" for most borderline patients and that if I can do this work, then so can most others. (Gunderson and Links 2014, p. ix)

We hope this book is a good enough start for you to provide early intervention for adolescents with BPD.

Chapter 9

Case Illustrations

THE CLINICAL VIGNETTES

in this chapter illustrate how to apply good psychiatric management for adolescents (GPM-A) principles in common clinical scenarios mental health professionals encounter. We offer decision points to give readers a chance to think through how they personally would respond before reading further. A nonexhaustive list of alternative responses to the decision points is then offered for the reader's consideration. To help with understanding which responses are more or less aligned with the GPM-A approach, the reader can rate which responses are helpful (scored as 1), possibly helpful but with continuing reservations (because the response depends on other considerations or because its effect seems unpredictable; scored as 2), and not helpful—or even harmful (scored as 3).

We encourage readers to think first about what they would do and why and reflect on their reactions to the different alternative responses. The spirit of GPM encourages clinicians to preserve their capacity to think independently and make reasoned decisions in realistically complex clinical situations where no one right answer exists. Rather, we emphasize that good clinical judgment depends on being aware of why you would take one course of action over another.

The discussion at the end of each case vignette examines the upsides and downsides of each alternative response from the GPM-A perspective, pointing readers toward relevant sections of the handbook where relevant GPM-A principles are presented. Most clinical decisions leave professionals in unresolved dilemmas that they can manage steadily using a coherent set of principles. You might disagree with suggested interventions. We encourage readers to take a position, understand how much it aligns with standards of care and evidence, and identify what GPM-A intervention would look like.

Case Vignette 1: Refusal and Subthreshold Borderline Personality Disorder (Carlos)

Chapters illustrated: Chapter 3 ("Making the Diagnosis and Providing Psychoeducation"), Chapter 4 ("Getting Started"), Chapter 6 ("Pharmacotherapy and Comorbidity"), and Chapter 7 ("Multimodal Treatments")

Teresa Carreño, M.D.

This vignette illustrates the management of subthreshold symptoms of borderline personality disorder (BPD) in a young teen who is refusing therapy. Although Carlos, because of his young age, is limited in his capacity to assent to treatment, treatment cannot be forced. This vignette illustrates a flexible way to approach Carlos and his family under these challenging circumstances. It also illustrates a diagnostic approach in young teens, in whom major psychiatric syndromes have not yet consolidated.

Alternative Responses at Decision Points

Choose 1=helpful; 2=possibly helpful, with continuing reservations; 3=not helpful—or even harmful

> Carlos is a 13-year-old adolescent boy sitting in your waiting room casting a dark glance at you from under his hoodie. Lisa, his mother, is sitting next to him and appears tense and burdened. Carlos was referred by his pediatrician after she found superficial cuts on his arms and thighs. He was re-

covering from a first acute episode of anorexia, having refused to eat after experiencing an emotional crisis at home about which he had refused to speak to anyone. Three months ago, after 2 full weeks of food refusal, he had been hospitalized for refeeding. His eating disorder had responded to a Maudsley approach, in which the family, with clinical and nutritional support, was actively involved in ensuring that he ate. His nutritional status had stabilized (body mass index improved from 17 to 18.4).

His mother explains that she had to force Carlos to come, that he did not want to talk to a therapist. Carlos purses his lips and averts his gaze. **(Decision point 1)**

1. Carlos is clearly an unwilling customer. In the waiting room, you are trying to decide how best to attempt to establish rapport:

   A. Implore Carlos to please come in and talk to you.
   B. Tell Lisa that Carlos is still a child and has to do what his mother says.
   C. Tell Lisa to come in first because Carlos does not seem to want to talk to you.
   D. Tell Carlos it is important for you to understand his point of view to see if you can be of help, then ask him whether he wants to talk to you alone first or whether he wants his mother to come in, too.

Carlos decides he wants his mother to come in with him. He quickly tells you that nothing is wrong with him and that he does not need therapy. He refuses to offer any further history, deferring to his mother for any further details.

Lisa relates that Carlos seemed fine until the school year was about to begin. The family had moved from another state and he was attending a new school away from his longtime childhood friends. After the move, Carlos withdrew more from his family and seemed quiet and sullen. After the crisis, he became belligerent with his parents and easily and intensely emotionally dysregulated, breaking objects and biting himself when he was very upset. Most recently, his pediatrician had discovered superficial cuts over Carlos's forearms and thighs. At school he was over-controlled and socially isolated and would not participate in class discussions. His grades were excellent. Carlos's self-harm and passive suicidal threats have been limited to episodes of mood dysregulation, which often were triggered by discord with his parents related to his eating and participating in treatment. He has not attempted suicide. **(Decision point 2)**

2. Given this limited information, what diagnoses would you consider, and which diagnostic priorities would you give them?

You meet with both parents and obtain a developmental history. Carlos suffered from intense separation anxiety in preschool and was a shy child. In kindergarten, he refused to speak to his teacher for months after he was

Diagnosis	Likelihood (1=yes, 2=possible, 3=no)	Priority (1=high, 2=medium, 3=low)
A. Borderline personality disorder		
B. Major depressive disorder		
C. Anorexia nervosa		
D. Bulimia nervosa		
E. Bipolar I disorder		
F. Bipolar II disorder		
G. Psychotic disorder		
H. PTSD		
I. Substance use disorder		

separated from his best friend. He finally adapted and did well academically. He typically has one best friend. He had been planning to attend his neighborhood middle school with his close friends before the family needed to move.

You complete the history and find that Carlos's BPD symptoms are subthreshold but nonetheless concerning. He self-harms, and he has difficulty regulating his intense anger. His introversion makes it difficult to directly assess his internal experience of interpersonal hypersensitivity; however, his symptoms are relational, triggered by discord with his parents. His mood is reactive. In your assessment, you also find that he met criteria for a major depressive episode when he had his crisis, but the major depressive symptoms have abated. Carlos remains sad and anxious more often than not. His anorexic symptoms continue to improve slowly. (**Decision point 3**)

3. What do you tell Carlos and his parents about his diagnosis and risk of BPD?

   A. You do not mention BPD to Carlos or his parents because he does not fully meet criteria.

   B. You disclose to Carlos and his parents that in addition to recovering from a major depressive episode and from an eating disorder, his current symptoms put him at risk of developing BPD.

   C. You disclose the risk of BPD to his parents, but you do not tell Carlos.

You disclose to Carlos and his parents that in addition to recovering from a major depressive episode and an eating disorder, he seems to be having a hard time with relationships since the move. When the family moved, he had to leave his old friends behind, and now he does not seem to be making new friends. You imagine he might feel a bit lonely in school. His closest relationships right now seem to be with his parents, and when he gets upset with them, his feelings become so intense that he can't think. His anger can feel too strong and out of control, and sometimes he hurts himself as a way of calming down. You tell Carlos and his parents that some teens can have problems in their relationships with others and even in their relationships with themselves, such as low self-confidence or not knowing who they are. This can put them at risk of developing more serious difficulties in the future such as BPD. These problems are treatable with psychotherapy that involves both Carlos and his parents, to help them help Carlos better. You recommend weekly sessions with Carlos and monthly sessions with his parents for 6 months, followed by a reevaluation. Carlos seems to listen and reluctantly agrees to meeting with you. The day of your first scheduled meeting with Carlos, he refuses to get out of the car, telling his mother that he does not need psychotherapy. Lisa calls from the car, clearly alarmed, asking you what to do. (**Decision point 4**)

4. At this juncture, how do you proceed?

    A. Tell Lisa to do her best to convince Carlos to come in and that you will wait for him for the full scheduled session time.

    B. Tell Lisa that Carlos must not have clearly agreed to the plan and that he needs to be in agreement for therapy to be helpful. Set up another meeting with Carlos and his parents where the goal will be collaborative planning that will necessitate his input.

    C. If Carlos refuses to come in, schedule a meeting with his parents to try to better understand Carlos's refusal.

    D. Go down to the car and try to help Lisa convince Carlos to come in for his psychotherapy appointment.

    E. Tell Lisa that if Carlos does not agree to psychotherapy, then it cannot be forced and she should return home and call when Carlos is ready to start therapy.

    You meet with Carlos's parents. They are visibly afraid and express feeling terrified that he cut himself after refusing his first appointment and refusing to speak with them. They slept in the same bed with him the previous night and left him home with his grandparents after hiding all the knives. You notice yourself feeling somewhat anxious; their worry feels a bit contagious. (**Decision point 5**)

5. What do you do now?

    A. You begin to inquire about suicide and question whether it is safe for Carlos to remain in an outpatient setting, given his self-harm and refusal to engage in treatment.

B. You tell Carlos's parents that it is essential for Carlos to participate in therapy if there is any chance that he will improve. You work with the parents to try to develop ways they can convince Carlos to attend the meetings using both arguments and behavioral reinforcers.

C. You notice your own discomfort as a signal of the high emotional intensity Carlos and his parents are trying to manage. You remind yourself that the cuts were superficial and establish that Carlos did not make suicidal threats. Your own reaction helps to inform you that the next step is to try to calm things down. You decide to work with Carlos's parents to do a chain analysis of what happened the day Carlos refused to come in.

D. Prescribe a selective serotonin reuptake inhibitor (SSRI) or an atypical antipsychotic to help Carlos with his mood dysregulation in an attempt to decrease his emotional intensity and self-harm.

When you run a chain analysis with Carlos's parents, you learn that they pulled him out of an after-school meeting for the school play at which he was intending to join the stage crew. You wonder to yourself whether your diagnostic disclosure to Carlos might have influenced his interest in becoming more involved with peers. Carlos had not told his parents about the meeting, and they felt the appointment with you was more important. Carlos was embarrassed to be pulled out and felt disappointed and misunderstood by his parents. When he refused to come to the therapy session, they felt helpless and angry. Emotions escalated, Carlos became dysregulated and cut himself, and his parents felt terrified.

As you slowly and empathically review what happened, Carlos's parents begin to realize how this situation got out of control. You note to yourself and to his parents that his participation in an organized group activity with peers (stage crew) is recommended and could help put him on track developmentally. You and his parents decide to meet biweekly for now because Carlos is refusing to meet with you.

In the next few weeks, you work with Carlos's parents to continue to look for relational triggers to his emotional dysregulation and threats of self-harm. You teach them to decrease their expressed emotional intensity and help them see that this helps Carlos regulate himself better. For example, you encourage them to make time to talk about neutral things with Carlos, such as his interest in plays, and to engage in pleasant family activities. You also help his parents focus on taking better care of themselves and getting together with friends and family. This helps to cool the emotional intensity at home (see Appendix D, "Guidelines for Families").

Even though Carlos continues to refuse to attend therapy meetings with you, his self-injurious behaviors stop. After his parents' discreet intervention at school, he is allowed to join the stage crew for the school play. Carlos seems a bit less sad and feels invested in the production. In their work with you, his parents are becoming better equipped to manage Carlos's relational sensitivity and intense emotional reactions.

Carlos seems to be doing very well. His grades are good, and he is relating more to his peers around the play. He has even begun participating more in class discussions. It seems as though he is fully back on track. The week before the play, however, his parents contact you. They heard Carlos screaming and crying in his room. He had bite marks on his arms. He felt angry and overwhelmed, and he couldn't say why. He told his parents he felt like dying, although he was not suicidal. (**Decision point 6**)

6. How do you respond?

    A. Express your concern to the parents that Carlos may be having a relapse of his depression. Suggest that they need to bring him in to see you so that you can evaluate for depression to see if medications can help.

    B. Tell the parents that this is likely a reaction to the play ending and also possibly a reaction to his significant improvement. Explain that improvement can be experienced as stressful in that Carlos might worry that people won't be as supportive anymore when he is better—and he might not even realize that this could be a worry he is having. Tell them it can help if they acknowledge his improvement and hard work and tell him that they are concerned about how stressful this might be for him. They might suggest he take things slowly and offer to help him come up with a plan to relieve his stress.

    C. Suggest to the parents that they offer to bring Carlos to their next meeting with you, that perhaps you can help them figure out how to help him feel better.

    D. Consider an SSRI or an atypical antipsychotic to help Carlos regulate his emotions better during this stressful time.

Carlos agrees to see you with his parents. In this session, it becomes clear that he felt very sad about the play ending. He would miss working with his friends and teachers and was worried that he might not feel as connected to them when it was over. With your help, he and his parents come up with a plan to attend a theater camp in the summer. Carlos does not want to meet with you regularly, but his parents feel more equipped to help him manage his distress, and Carlos is more willing to use your help should he feel he needs it.

Discussion

1. Carlos is clearly an unwilling customer. In the waiting room, you are trying to decide how best to attempt to establish rapport:

A. Implore Carlos to please come in and talk to you. [2] Carlos is already tense, so imploring him without reasoning is likely to increase his tension and his unwillingness. Carlos has never met you, and you do not know why he is refusing to talk to a therapist. The first step will need to involve better understanding his concern and his mother's tension and worry.

B. Tell Lisa that Carlos is still a child and has to do what his mother says. [3] Calling Carlos a "child" and attempting to force him to participate against his will would be experienced as invalidating and controlling. Carlos's mother already brought him to your waiting room with a great deal of effort. Carlos is expressing his negative feelings about being there. This approach would likely be difficult to repair, particularly because rapport has not yet been established.

C. Tell Lisa to come in first because Carlos does not seem to want to talk to you. [2] Quickly asking Carlos's mother to come in first bypasses acknowledging and showing interest in Carlos's expressed concern. He is likely to feel unseen and dismissed. If he agrees, he is likely to feel very uncomfortable waiting alone while his mother speaks about him to someone he does not know. It is possible that he will prefer to come in with his mother rather than to wait alone.

D. Tell Carlos it is important for you to understand his point of view to see if you can be of help, then ask him whether he wants to talk to you alone first or whether he wants his mother to come in, too. [1] Expressing interest in Carlos's perspective and allowing him to influence your perspective demonstrates a collaborative and validating approach. You are also allowing Carlos to participate in deciding the structure of your first meeting with him, respecting his sense of autonomy and agency.

2. Given this limited information, what diagnoses would you consider, and which diagnostic priorities would you give them?

Diagnosis	Likelihood (1=yes, 2=possible, 3=no)	Priority (1=high, 2=medium, 3=low)	Comments
A. Borderline personality disorder (BPD)	2	1	Carlos shows externalizing and internalizing symptoms.
B. Major depressive disorder	2	2	
C. Anorexia nervosa	1	2	Carlos is eating, and his body mass index is almost typical.
D. Bulimia nervosa	2	2	
E. Bipolar I disorder	2	1	Carlos demonstrates no mania or grandiosity (Geller and Luby 1997).
F. Bipolar II disorder	2	3	
G. Psychotic disorder	3	1	Carlos has no psychotic symptoms.
H. PTSD	2	2	You must obtain a trauma history before making a PTSD diagnosis.
I. Substance use disorder	2	2	You should obtain a history. Substance use disorder is a primary diagnosis if it is causing dysfunction and should be addressed within BPD treatment.

3. What do you tell Carlos and his parents about his diagnosis and risk of BPD?

    A. You do not mention BPD to Carlos or his parents because he does not fully meet criteria. [3] It has been found that in risk-taking or self-harming teens, patients with three symptoms of BPD showed similar impairment in quality of life as those meeting full criteria for BPD (Kaess et al. 2017). Carlos demonstrates a combination of internalizing and externalizing symptoms, which might suggest a BPD diagnosis (Sharp and Fonagy 2015). His current level of morbidity can interfere with his normal development in adolescence. Early intervention could prevent substantial morbidity in the future. For these reasons, his parents need to be informed.

    B. You disclose to Carlos and his parents that in addition to recovering from a major depressive episode and from an eating disorder, his current symptoms put him at risk of developing BPD. [1] Carlos's residual symptoms are part of the symptom picture of BPD, and although he does not fully meet criteria, he has three symptoms. It is useful to inform Carlos and his parents that although he is shy and reserved, he has always been a person of intense feelings, and because he is very private, he can be difficult to read, making it more likely that he will be misunderstood. This intensity and not being accurately understood can predispose a person to developing BPD, and this can be treated.

    C. You disclose the risk of BPD to his parents, but you do not tell Carlos. [2] In adolescence, diagnostic disclosure varies depending on the patient's age and family circumstances. For younger teens, it is often helpful to address the diagnosis first with parents, disclosing to the teen once parents have understood and accepted the diagnosis.

4. At this juncture, how do you proceed?

    A. Tell Lisa to do her best to convince Carlos to come in and that you will wait for him for the full scheduled session time. [2] You are giving Lisa and Carlos the opportunity to try to work out his refusal with each other. The main difficulty is that Lisa sounds alarmed. Their high level of emotional intensity might be making it difficult for either of them to think clearly at that moment, and both may not yet be equipped with the skills needed to manage the situation. Reassuring Lisa might be helpful.

    B. Tell Lisa that Carlos must not have clearly agreed to the plan and that he needs to be in agreement for therapy to be helpful. Set up another meeting with Carlos and his parents where the goal will be collaborative planning that will necessitate his input. [2] Before you meet with Carlos and his parents together, Lisa's alarm should be addressed and diminished and her curiosity piqued. At age 13, Carlos's developmental capacity to assent to therapy is limited. By the same token, therapy cannot be forced. Did Carlos initially agree to psychotherapy—was he even informed? If he did agree to therapy, why does he not want to come in today? Did he know he had an appointment? Is he reacting to an unrelated disappointment? Is Carlos averse to psychotherapy for other reasons? It will first be necessary to understand the nature of Carlos's refusal in order to decide how to proceed. There are not enough data at this juncture to know whether Carlos has not agreed with the plan.

C. If Carlos refuses to come in, schedule a meeting with his parents to try to better understand Carlos's refusal. [1] Understanding what is driving Carlos's behavior internally is essential, and it is also essential to understand how his mother is understanding and experiencing his refusal to come into the session. Only with these data can the next step be determined.

D. Go down to the car and try to help Lisa convince Carlos to come in for his psychotherapy appointment. [2] Going down to the car might be helpful, but not with the intent of convincing Carlos. Rather, you could try to help decrease the level of emotional intensity. The first step is to try to understand how Carlos and his mother are experiencing this moment and what thoughts and feelings are driving Carlos's behavior and her reaction to it. This understanding will help inform how to proceed.

E. Tell Lisa that if Carlos does not agree to psychotherapy, then it cannot be forced and she should return home and call when Carlos is ready to start therapy. [3] This decision leaves both Carlos and his mother unsupported, while what is driving Carlos's refusal has yet to be understood. The appropriate next step involves trying to understand what is happening internally for Carlos and for his mother that is resulting in his refusal and in her sense of alarm. Even if Carlos refuses psychotherapy, it is clear that his parents need support.

5. What do you do now?

A. You begin to inquire about suicide and question whether it is safe for Carlos to remain in an outpatient setting, given his self-harm and refusal to engage in treatment. [3] Carlos's cuts are superficial and there is no evidence of suicidality. His symptoms had been improving. His parents' willingness to engage in family work creates an opening to help Carlos, if not directly, then indirectly by helping his parents learn to understand him and manage his symptoms more effectively.

B. You tell Carlos's parents that it is essential for Carlos to participate in therapy if there is any chance that he will improve. You work with the parents to try to develop ways they can convince Carlos to attend the meetings using both arguments and behavioral reinforcers. [2] It would likely help if Carlos were willing to engage in therapy; however, the emotional thermometer at home is too hot at this moment for anyone to think clearly (even you are feeling a bit challenged). Presenting his parents with this demand at this time would likely make them feel even more worried. It would be best first to decrease the level of emotional intensity prior to addressing how to help Carlos consider returning.

C. You notice your own discomfort as a signal of the high emotional intensity Carlos and his parents are trying to manage. You remind yourself that the cuts were superficial and establish that Carlos did not make suicidal threats. Your own reaction helps to inform you that the next step is to try to calm things down. You decide to work with Carlos's parents to do a chain analysis of what happened the day Carlos refused to come in. [1] You do not know what upset Carlos prior to refusing to come into your session. A careful review of what preceded the situation, with a focus on interpersonal triggers, will likely make his behavior more understandable to you and to his parents. This very process will help model for his parents a curious stance as they try to better understand the underpinnings of Carlos's emotions and behaviors.

D. Prescribe an SSRI or an atypical antipsychotic to help Carlos with his mood dysregulation in an attempt to decrease his emotional intensity and self-harm. [3] Sometimes, medications can be useful as an adjuvant to psychotherapy (see Chapter 6). However, is unlikely that Carlos is going to agree to take a medication at this juncture, and adding another demand will likely not be helpful at this time. Also, it is early in the process to prescribe medication because a frame of treatment has not yet been established. Pharmacotherapy at this point risks establishing unrealistic expectations as to the effectiveness of medications in treating Carlos's BPD symptoms.

6. How do you respond?

    A. Express your concern to the parents that Carlos may be having a re-lapse of his depression. Suggest that they need to bring him in to see you so that you can evaluate for depression to see if medications can help. [3] Carlos has been improving steadily. Given his history, his sudden and intense distress is most likely a reaction to a relational disruption or threat. This would best be managed by trying to understand what triggered his reaction. Assuming a depressive relapse too quickly could lead to missing the relational triggers, possible misdiagnosis, and iatrogenic pharmacological treatment.

    B. Tell the parents that this is likely a reaction to the play ending and also possibly a reaction to his significant improvement. Explain that improvement can be experienced as stressful in that Carlos might worry that people won't be as supportive anymore when he is better—and he might not even realize that this could be a worry he is having. Tell them it can help if they acknowledge his improvement and hard work and tell him that they are concerned about how stressful this might be for him. They might suggest he take things slowly and offer to help him come up with a plan to relieve his stress. [1] In patients with BPD, progress can evoke fears of abandonment (see Appendix D). It is helpful if treaters and family members do not express too much excitement about progress, and you should caution against moving too fast.

    C. Suggest to the parents that they offer to bring Carlos to their next meeting with you, that perhaps you can help them figure out how to help him feel better. [1] In view of Carlos's improvement and the improved relationship with his parents, it could be of benefit to invite Carlos to use your help now that he is experiencing distress. Should he accept, you could become another direct resource for him when he does not feel well. He might be more open at this time because his initial refusal seemed to be a reaction to having felt forced by his parents.

    D. Consider an SSRI or an atypical antipsychotic to help Carlos regulate his emotions better during this stressful time. [2] Carlos is intensely dysphoric and dysregulated. A limited course of medication might be helpful (see Chapter 6). However, before making this decision, it would be useful to better understand and address the triggers of his distress. If Carlos does not respond to these interventions or if his symptoms do not remit or they intensify, adjunctive psycho-pharmacological intervention might be of benefit.

Case Vignette 2: Forming a Therapeutic Alliance (Evelyn)

Chapters illustrated: Chapter 3 ("Making the Diagnosis and Providing Psychoeducation"), Chapter 4 ("Getting Started"), Chapter 5 ("Managing Suicidality and Nonsuicidal Self-Injury"), Chapter 6 ("Pharmacotherapy and Comorbidity"), and Chapter 7 ("Multimodal Treatments")

Eduardo Martinho Jr., M.D., Ph.D.

This vignette involves an adolescent, Evelyn, who is struggling with school absenteeism, self-harm, suicidal ideation, and alcohol abuse. Her family environment is highly volatile and unstable, with rigid notions of sexual orientation. The vignette describes efforts to form a therapeutic alliance with Evelyn and her parents, to deal effectively with confidentiality issues, and to remain active but not reactive in the face of difficult situations. Additionally, it underscores the importance of providing BPD diagnostic disclosure in a way that reduces stigma and promotes family engagement and reduction of ineffective interventions such as polypharmacy and recurrent hospitalizations.

Alternative Responses at Decision Points

Choose 1=helpful; 2=possibly helpful, with continuing reservations; 3=not helpful—or even harmful

> Evelyn is a 17-year-old Filipino American girl living in California with her parents, Anton (47 years old, lawyer) and Lucia (39 years old, nurse). She is referred to you by a primary care doctor and presents with depressive symptoms, panic attacks, and self-harm. She has been taking sertraline 50 mg and alprazolam 0.5 mg as needed for 2 weeks.
>
> Lucia recalls that, throughout elementary school in San Diego, Evelyn was a very sensitive child, obedient and active in church, with good grades but a lot of anxiety and no close friends in school. When Evelyn was 8 years old, she began describing herself as a very ugly person, saying there was no way that other people could possibly like her. She feels this way primarily because of a large birthmark that covers most of her face and because her father is often too busy with work to spend time with the family. Anton also struggles with a severe gambling addiction that put the family in debt, about which he and Lucia often argue loudly in front of Evelyn. Whenever this happens, Evelyn runs to her bedroom, "her safe place," and at age 11 she began to self-harm at least monthly to cope with her overwhelming feelings.

When Evelyn was 14, her family moved to San Francisco, where she became very connected to three friends in her new school. She began showing more impulsive behaviors, yelling at her parents and hiding an intense romantic relationship from them for 3 months when she was dating a girl from her school who was 3 years older. Her parents were focused on academic grades and strict religious values, so Evelyn was not allowed to go to parties or to hang out with friends during the weekends. However, she sneaked out of the house regularly to meet up with friends, get drunk, and sometimes race each other down the highway late at night. She says, "It makes me feel free—like I don't have a care in the world."

As the months passed, Evelyn became less and less connected to her church and her parents. When she was 16, she discovered that her mother was having an affair. During a discussion with her parents, she yelled that they were hypocritical, that her father was an addict, and that her mother was a cheating slut, revealing her mother's secret. Following this angry outburst, Evelyn's parents decided to separate, and Evelyn and Lucia moved back to San Diego. Evelyn felt responsible for this separation and increased her self-harm as a way to cope with feeling rejected. Despite being in deep financial trouble, Anton has never sought treatment and continues to go to casinos, convinced it is the only way to regain the money he has lost and make it up to his family.

After moving back to San Diego, Evelyn had trouble adapting to her new school, was absent on many occasions, got poor grades, and struggled to make friends. She missed her friends in San Francisco and called them many times a day until they got uncomfortable with it and asked her to stop calling. The only person she talks to in school is a girl, Laura, to whom she is very attracted. Evelyn has never had sex, and she defines her sexual orientation as pansexual. She is very afraid of being punished if her parents discover her sexual orientation.

In the past month, Evelyn has been drinking more and more—even when not with peers—and her self-harm behavior has increased to at least three times a week, often occurring when she is drunk alone. At first, Lucia said that she was just trying to make a scene, but when Evelyn showed her the bleeding from a deep self-inflicted cut on her arm, Lucia became desperate and took Evelyn to the hospital. A suture was needed for the wound, and the clinician referred Evelyn to a psychiatrist. The only available appointment with a psychiatrist was in 1 month, so Lucia made an earlier appointment with a general practitioner, who did not explain anything about Evelyn's diagnosis. The general practitioner asked that Evelyn stay out of school for 2 weeks, prescribed sertraline 50 mg and alprazolam 0.5 mg as needed, and referred her to you.

In this first session, Evelyn appears vigilant, intelligent, and desperate for help. Initially, she is very worried about what you will say to her mother (her father is not present). **(Decision point 1)**

1. In this first session, regarding confidentiality, you should

   A. Tell Evelyn that as her clinician, you know that the only way to stay connected to her is by keeping all material that is sensitive for her private.

B. Tell Evelyn that, considering her suicidal ideation and that there are severe communication problems in her family, you must help her to be frank about everything with her parents and that she will find relief in doing so.

C. Tell Evelyn that as her therapist, you are legally responsible for her safety, so by necessity you have the final say on what is shared with her parents and what is not.

D. Tell Evelyn that keeping confidentiality about sensitive material in therapy is a priority. Describe your goal as being able to collaborate with her on defining what is private and what her parents may need to know. Whenever possible, you will plan with her how, when, and to whom the disclosure will take place. The only exception to this would be in situations where her physical safety, related to suicide or self-harm, are at severe risk and the two of you are unable to find a way to agree on how to involve her parents.

You feel emotionally connected to Evelyn. She tells you that this is the first time someone has really listened to her instead of trying to fix her. She feels that being in the same room with her mother talking about these issues will be very complicated for her, and she asks if you could talk to her mother alone, without Evelyn being present. You agree that this would be the best option. You ask her if, after talking to her mother, you can spend a few minutes discussing her medications and a viable treatment frame. She agrees with you.

Lucia complains about Evelyn's behavior, saying that she is walking on eggshells with her daughter, afraid that she could hurt herself again. Lucia says she recognizes she is harsh with her, but that she does it with her daughter's best interests at heart. She asks you about Evelyn's diagnosis. **(Decision point 2)**

2. In this first appointment, what is the most effective way to address the diagnosis?

A. Insist you must first talk to Anton because you think that his gambling addiction and neglecting his family for work may have created a severe emotional trauma for Evelyn.

B. Explain that Evelyn has BPD and provide psychoeducation about it, focusing on the presence of an invalidating environment as one of the causes for this disorder.

C. Focus on the model of interpersonal hypersensitivity and how it explains Evelyn's emotional and behavioral shifts. Also, it can explain Lucia's tendency to be harsh. Emphasize how a joint effort from the mental health clinician, school, and family can be the most effective tool to treat this condition.

D. The focus in this moment should be to target pharmacologically depressive symptoms, and if you succeed in this goal, there is a high possibility of remission of the interpersonal dysfunction and the suicide risk.

Lucia agrees to bring Anton to the next session. You bring Evelyn back and talk briefly about the treatment frame. You will see her weekly and talk to her parents at least monthly. You give her the number for the hospital paging system and explain confidentiality and its limits. You also explain that although she is not in crisis now, it is important to develop a safety plan proactively for managing moments where she may have urges to self-harm or suicidal thoughts. You discuss the medications that she is currently taking and schedule another appointment for the following week. (**Decision point 3**)

3. Initially, how would you manage Evelyn's medications?

A. Considering this is the first session, tell Evelyn's parents that you do not feel comfortable making changes in her medication and that you will tackle this issue properly in the next session.

B. Ask Evelyn about her use of alprazolam, explain your concerns about the relationship between benzodiazepines and impulsivity, and work with her to find a way to discontinue the medication.

C. Taking into account the high comorbidity between BPD and bipolar disorder, reduce the use of antidepressants and start a mood stabilizer.

D. Ask Evelyn about what happened regarding suicidal thoughts after initiating the use of sertraline. Request that she monitor these thoughts during the coming week and let you know if they get worse. Talk about the black box warning; although suicidal thoughts are not common, it is important for everyone to help in monitoring them.

At her second appointment, Evelyn tells you that she has noticed that although her mother has kept her usual emotional distance, she seems calmer and more at ease. Evelyn has not had any episode of self-harm since the first appointment (4 days ago), but she spent most of her time locked in her room watching TV, and she did get drunk alone in her room. She tells you that she drinks because it helps her momentarily forget about her strong feelings of emptiness and that she feels she has no idea who she really is. She sometimes wonders if she really exists. She says that although she is not planning suicide, she sees it as a possible solution for her emotional pain. She believes in the possibility of reducing her suicidal thoughts and rumination but feels hopeless that any medication could ever relieve her feelings of emptiness. Evelyn has been out of school for almost 4 weeks, and whenever she tries to do anything related to school, she gets panicky. She misses talking to Laura, although they are texting. She expresses her attraction to Laura and feels optimistic that Laura may return her feelings. Although Evelyn fears returning to school, she also dreads the possibility of needing to repeat the academic year. (**Decision point 4**)

4. Regarding Evelyn's school absenteeism, you should

   A. Focus on the remission of Evelyn's residual depressive symptoms, alcohol use, and high levels of anxiety before she attempts to go back to school. The decline of efficacy in executive functioning caused by these symptoms could compromise her academic performance, leading to unbearable feelings of shame.

   B. Tell Evelyn that going back to school is the only way to achieve recovery, and it is worth paying the price of getting panicky to achieve it.

   C. Tell Evelyn that considering her emotional pain and the necessity of attending school, you will work with her and her parents on alternatives such as therapeutic boarding schools, home schooling, and online schools.

   D. Tell Evelyn that you and her family will have to find a balance between empathy for her emotional pain and the need to gradually return to school for her recovery. You will work with her family to get in contact with her school counselor to make sure that there is a feasible plan for her gradual return to school.

You start working with Evelyn on the crisis plan and a chain analysis about her most recent alcohol use. It is clear she drinks alcohol to attenuate her feelings of social inferiority and inadequacy. Also, after a thorough assessment using the DSM-5 criteria for BPD (American Psychiatric Association 2013), you establish and discuss a BPD diagnosis with Evelyn and Lucia, using an accessible language. After this conversation, you realize that both Evelyn and Lucia now have more realistic expectations from medications and a richer understanding about the negative impacts of prolonged hospitalization. You use the diagnostic disclosure to emphasize the importance of empathetic communication and regular attendance to the sessions (for both Evelyn and her parents). Finally, you reinforce the necessity of finding a balance in helping Evelyn to "make sense" of her emotional pain and her interpersonal hypersensitivity, with the goal of getting back to school, a crucial step for BPD recovery. She loves using a phone application that guides her through coping skills and finds that it really helps her stop and think before drinking or cutting.

Lucia tells you that Anton will not be able to attend the coming sessions because he has just started work at a new law firm, but he will be available in about a month. Lucia also tells you that she has already contacted Evelyn's school counselor, who is eager to call you. The following week, the school counselor, with your help, develops a plan for Evelyn's return to school. The counselor tells you that she appreciates your suggestions and that she appreciated reading the material you recommended to her (www.projectairstrategy.org/content/groups/public/@web/@project-air/documents/doc/uow262247.pdf). Evelyn stayed sober and was able to attend classes 3 days in the past week (although she had to return home early on 2 of those days), and you brainstorm strategies with her to deal with her anxiety.

The day before your fifth session, Lucia went through Evelyn's phone without her knowledge and found flirtatious text messages she had written to Laura. Lucia became extremely angry and confronted Evelyn, telling her, "You would cause me much less pain if you were pregnant. I did not raise you to be a lesbian!" She took Evelyn's cell phone from her. Evelyn cut herself, cried all night, and experienced a marked increase in suicidal thoughts. She cries during the session as well. (**Decision points 5 and 6**)

5. Regarding the family discussion Lucia and Evelyn had yesterday, what should you do?

   A. Protect Evelyn, making clear to Lucia that looking at Evelyn's cell phone behind her back is very inappropriate behavior; that homophobia is a crime; and that if she continues this homophobic behavior toward Evelyn, you will report it to a child protective agency.

   B. To decrease conflict, ask Evelyn to not fight back against Lucia because doing so would only add fuel to the fire, then teach her some distress tolerance skills.

   C. Demonstrate a strong commitment to understanding each of their points of view about this conflict. Ask them what attitudes they expect from you and then work on finding a balance between protecting Evelyn and keeping your therapeutic alliance with Lucia.

   D. Ask Lucia what possible outcomes she thinks are likely to occur after forbidding Evelyn to use her cell phone.

   E. Work with Lucia to find a way of balancing her religious values with the necessity of all the family members respecting each other even when they have a disagreement. You could also say this balance is syntonic with the key religious values of respect, mercy, and compassion.

   F. Tell Lucia that sexual orientation might be fluid in many adolescents and that Lucia's behavior of harsh punishment could reinforce the outcome she is trying to prevent.

6. With regard to the increase in suicidal thoughts reported by Evelyn, what should you do?

A. Considering that Evelyn has expressed an increase in suicidal ideation and that a change in Lucia's stance will take some time, recommend that Evelyn be admitted to an inpatient psychiatric facility.

B. Assess the danger of the situation, differentiating suicidal ideation from true suicidal intention.

C. Ask Evelyn whether this increase in suicidal ideation is related to experiences of rejection she felt regarding Lucia's reaction.

D. Ask Lucia and Evelyn to sign a written contract that Evelyn will not self-harm or kill herself and that Lucia will not demonstrate judgmental homophobic behaviors.

E. After talking about ways that you will work with Lucia to improve Evelyn's safety, discuss how Evelyn can help herself when she is in situations or emotional states that lead to self-harm or an increase in her suicidal ideation.

F. Explain to Lucia that punishment as a response to sexual orientation is correlated with suicide. Then say to Lucia that you want to find a way to respect her family's religious values and at the same time protect Evelyn's life, asking how she could help you to do so.

G. Prescribe quetiapine 25 mg daily to decrease the risk of suicidal behaviors.

H. Access Evelyn's crisis plan again and work with her on skills that could be added to it.

I. Ask Evelyn if there is anyone in her family who is more supportive about sexual orientation who could be included in her treatment to help her.

J. Tell Lucia that you are very concerned that Evelyn is without her cell phone: "Remaining without a cell phone could seriously jeopardize the execution of our crisis plan, which includes calling me or other supports to help her. Let's find parameters for its use that both of you can agree on right now."

After your intervention, you feel Lucia understands the risks of a rejecting or punitive response to Evelyn's sexual orientation. Lucia has agreed to work with you in the coming weeks to deal with the issue in a more effective way. Evelyn is very grateful for the way you have responded to this situation, helping the family through a crisis without hospitalization. Two weeks later, Anton finally attends a session. During this interview, you find that he has severe depressive symptomatology in addition to his gambling problems, and he agrees to be referred to another mental health professional. You work with Evelyn on ways to maintain her own sobriety (e.g., joining a dialectical behavior therapy [DBT] skills group, throwing away hidden alcohol and her fake ID), as well as to improve her school and social environments. Evelyn researches different extracurricular options so she can have more structure. She is very interested in joining her high school theater program.

You are 15 minutes late for Evelyn's session today. You did not let her know you would be late in advance, and she looks irritated and upset, but she does not say anything. (**Decision point 7**)

7. Regarding your late arrival to this appointment, you should

A. Apologize for being late, recognize that Evelyn is right to be upset, and ask her forgiveness for what you did. Tell her that after causing her such pain, you are feeling guilty, and you feel the current session is a lost cause. Then reschedule a new appointment free of charge as soon as possible.

B. Apologize for being late, then use this event as an opportunity to explain how interpersonal hypersensitivity might have contributed to her intense emotional response toward you.

C. Say you are sad and sorry for being late and that if you were in her shoes, you would feel irritated and upset. Ask Evelyn to describe what she is feeling at this moment and work with her to find the most effective way to handle this situation.

D. Apologize for being late and explain with genuine emotion the pressing demands that caused you to be late for this session.

E. Tell Evelyn that you notice she is upset with you and that this is fair because you were late. However, considering that you are not usually late, she should demonstrate more empathy for you, just as you did when she was late for some appointments in the past.

In the next session, both of you get to the session on time, and you are very curious to know if Evelyn enrolled in the school theater program. She tells you she has and shares that she has not been spending as much time with the friends she used to sneak out and get drunk with because she is forming new friendships in the theater program and is busy trying to catch up on school. You take this as a good sign that she is progressing toward some of her goals. However, these new expectations and friendships have given Evelyn a resurgence of overwhelming anxiety that she is struggling to manage without drinking to calm her down, so you know there is still more work to do together to keep her on the path of improvement.

Discussion

1. In this first session, regarding confidentiality, you should

    A. Tell Evelyn that as her clinician, you know that the only way to stay connected to her is by keeping all material that is sensitive for her private. [3] If you do not say anything about the limits of confidentiality, you may encounter an irreparable rupture of the therapeutic alliance if you need to break confidentiality in the context of safety concerns. Unconditional confidentiality is outside the legal boundaries of confidentiality protection. Being explicit about good standards of care at the initiation of treatment helps frame the roles and goals of the treatment relationship. You can take note of the connected state Lucia is in and make use of it to broker an alliance while remaining realistic about the limits of your ability to be exclusively on her side.

    B. Tell Evelyn that, considering her suicidal ideation and that there are severe communication problems in her family, you must help her to be frank about everything with her parents and that she will find relief in doing so. [3] Most adolescents will not disclose the very behaviors that bring them to treatment if they believe their parents will be notified, which can make it more difficult to make use of treatment. Developing of independence from parents is an important task of adolescence, and protection of confidentiality is essential to this process. Clinicians can assure adolescents that what they discuss in therapy will be kept private except when not doing so could represent a serious threat to their safety.

    C. Tell Evelyn that, as her therapist, you are legally responsible for her safety, so by necessity you have the final say on what is shared with her parents and what is not. [3] This authoritarian approach will not go over well with adolescents, who are at a developmental stage where they are growing in independence. This would not be a good start to building a trusting, collaborative therapeutic alliance and runs the risk of Evelyn not speaking with you openly because of fears that you will report everything she says to her parents.

    D. Tell Evelyn that keeping confidentiality about sensitive material in therapy is a priority. Describe your goal as being able to collaborate with her on defining what is private and what her parents may need to know. Whenever possible, you will plan with her how, when, and to whom the disclosure will take place. The only exception to this would be in situations where her physical safety, related to suicide or self-harm, is at severe risk and the two of you are unable to find a way to agree on how to involve her parents. [1] Using this approach, you are trying to create a balancing act between ensuring some level of confidentiality, which will lead to greater honesty and openness, and the need to help Evelyn's parents protect her safety. This approach also puts Evelyn in a more accountable position in the treatment.

2. In this first appointment, what is the most effective way to address the diagnosis?

   A. Insist you must first talk to Anton because you think that his gambling addiction and neglecting his family for work may have created a severe emotional trauma for Evelyn. [3] Even if parental dynamics are contributing to the etiology of Evelyn's problems, a confrontational approach in the first appointment may prevent you from creating an even and structured alliance with both Evelyn and her parents. In addition, your focus on her father's failings might put Evelyn in a situation that could reinforce her feelings of shame and guilt. Of course, you should not ignore Anton's gambling behaviors, but it is important to first try to develop a therapeutic alliance with Evelyn's parents before tackling this issue.

   B. Explain that Evelyn has BPD and provide psychoeducation about it, focusing on the presence of an invalidating environment as one of the causes for this disorder. [2] Disclosing the BPD diagnosis might be helpful in facilitating a treatment alliance. However, at this juncture, where Evelyn's environment is charged with emotional tension, disclosing the diagnosis in this first appointment may elevate tensions. Taking more time to talk to Evelyn, Lucia, and Anton separately would help you be clearer on each of their views of the problem without the reactivity between family members taking center stage.

   C. Focus on the model of interpersonal hypersensitivity and how it explains Evelyn's emotional and behavioral shifts. Also, it can explain Lucia's tendency to be harsh. Emphasize how a joint effort from the mental health clinician, school, and family can be the most effective tool to treat this condition. [1] Focusing first on interpersonal hypersensitivity is a descriptive starting point in explaining the oscillations in Evelyn's behaviors and Lucia's responses. At the same time, it can inform how the treatment works, and it underscores the importance of family and school engagement to improve Evelyn's symptomatology. In subsequent sessions, when you feel that disclosing BPD will facilitate treatment alliance, you can do so.

D. The focus in this moment should be to target pharmacologically depressive symptoms, and if you succeed in this goal, there is a high possibility of remission of the interpersonal dysfunction and the suicide risk. [3] Even if Evelyn has depression, an excessive focus on a pharmacological approach can induce passivity and take attention away from the family conflicts, which can aggravate Evelyn's symptoms. Medications are a secondary strategy in treatment for BPD. You do not want Lucia and Evelyn to think that medications are likely to solve her clear problems; rather, you want them to consider the psychological and social sources of Evelyn's symptoms.

3. Initially, how would you manage Evelyn's medications?

A. Considering this is the first session, tell Evelyn's parents that you do not feel comfortable making changes in Evelyn's medication and that you will tackle this issue properly in the next session. [3] Keeping the as-needed use of alprazolam might disinhibit Evelyn and can increase self-harm. Therefore, even in a first appointment, it is necessary to gather information about how all medications came to be prescribed and their effects on Evelyn. You should also provide psychoeducation about the limitations of their effectiveness for BPD.

B. Ask Evelyn about her use of alprazolam, explain your concerns about the relationship between benzodiazepines and impulsivity, and work with her to find a way to discontinue the medication. [1] This demonstrates your concerns about benzodiazepines and puts Evelyn in a more active role.

C. Taking into account the high comorbidity between BPD and bipolar disorder, reduce the use of antidepressants and start a mood stabilizer. [3] You do not have enough data in this case to make a diagnosis of bipolar disorder. Even if Evelyn does have bipolar disorder, prescribing a mood stabilizer during the first appointment, without a thorough health evaluation and identification of acute medical problems, would be premature diagnostic certainty without adequate information.

D. Ask Evelyn about what happened regarding suicidal thoughts after initiating the use of sertraline. Request that she monitor these thoughts during the coming week and let you know if they get worse. Talk about the black box warning; although suicidal thoughts are not common, it is important for everyone to help in monitoring them. [1] With this approach, you can detect whether Evelyn has developed any emotional "connection" with the medication and can use the monitoring of sertraline as a step toward creating a collaborative approach to working with the family.

4. Regarding Evelyn's school absenteeism, you should

A. Focus on the remission of Evelyn's residual depressive symptoms, alcohol use, and high levels of anxiety before she attempts to go back to school. The decline of efficacy in executive functioning caused by these symptoms could compromise her academic performance, leading to unbearable feelings of shame. [3] If you wait until her depressive symptoms are in remission to reintegrate Evelyn into her school, it will be difficult to provide opportunities to escape stressors at home and make progress in restoring her roles as student and friend at school. The more delayed her return to school activities, the harder it will be to achieve it. Sheltering Evelyn from usual demands as a solution to her stress sensitivity can reinforce passivity and avoidance. This is an unintended way to promote an iatrogenic treatment, when escape rather than adaptation becomes the solution to her problems, and over time this can contribute to the chronicity of her symptoms.

B. Tell Evelyn that going back to school is the only way to achieve recovery, and it is worth paying the price of getting panicky to achieve it. [2] The problem with this approach is that it puts all the weight of going back to school on Evelyn's shoulders, minimizing the challenges she will face with her return to school. Forcing this message may press independence in a way that will continue to cause Evelyn to feel threatened and to stay in a state of anger and self-harm.

C. Tell Evelyn that considering her emotional pain and the necessity of attending school, you will work with her and her parents on alternatives such as therapeutic boarding schools, home schooling, and online schools. [3] This plan is too focused on Evelyn's emotional pain and creates environmental change as a definitive solution prior to a trial of supporting a return to a more familiar setting. Before thinking about these options, you first have to work with Evelyn's family and school to gradually reintroduce her to the school environment in a reasonable and feasible way.

D. Tell Evelyn that you and her family will have to find a balance between empathy for her emotional pain and the need to gradually return to school for her recovery. You will work with her family to get in contact with her school counselor to make sure that there is a feasible plan for her gradual return to school. [1] You should find a balance between recognizing Evelyn's emotional pain and addressing the necessity of not delaying her return to school. For instance, you should contact the school to develop a safety and support plan that helps Evelyn and her school deal effectively with the struggles of her return to school. It is important to send the message that Evelyn's job as a student requires both independence and support rather than dichotomizing them. Adding an educational consultant to this process of returning to school can be very helpful.

5. Regarding the family discussion Lucia and Evelyn had yesterday, what should you do?

A. Protect Evelyn, making clear to Lucia that looking at Evelyn's cell phone behind her back is very inappropriate behavior; that homophobia is a crime; and that if she continues this homophobic behavior toward Evelyn, you will report it to a child protective agency. [2] Clinicians aim to provide an inclusive and respectful environment for patients by supporting their choices and being open and curious about their developing sexual and gender identity, but providing a forum for families to begin to discuss these aspects of development productively can be short-circuited by judgmental evaluations of patients or family members. Before confronting Lucia, it is important to make sure that you invest time in a thoughtful conversation, listening to her concerns and asking about her feelings. This will enable a more robust alliance with Lucia so you can help her be more supportive in your shared aim of effective treatment of Evelyn's BPD-related problems. Quick fix solutions are often inadequate. An aggressive confrontation may cause more harm for Evelyn's welfare than good by continuing a polarizing dynamic.

B. To decrease conflict, ask Evelyn to not fight back against Lucia because doing so would only add fuel to the fire, then teach her some distress tolerance skills. [2] This can reinforce beliefs that her sexuality is wrong and that it should be kept hidden. It is important to Evelyn to hear from you explicit statements of support for her sexual rights and validation of the painful harm of social prejudices. Before working with Evelyn on skills to deal with Lucia, you have to make clear to Evelyn that you want to accept her choices. Let her know that you are going to help her family have a more productive dialogue so they can feel comfortable with her choices, and you need to rely on her to work with you to demonstrate her ability to cope effectively.

C. Demonstrate a strong commitment to understanding each of their points of view about this conflict. Ask them what attitudes they expect from you and then work on finding a balance between protecting Evelyn and keeping your therapeutic alliance with Lucia. [1] In fact, helping Lucia change her behaviors, which are reinforced by custom, habit, and culture, will involve focusing first on understanding, respect, and compassion instead of recrimination and shame-inducing lectures. You should talk about Evelyn's coming out as a process, highlighting that even if some people react negatively, these attitudes may change over time.

D. Ask Lucia what possible outcomes she thinks are likely to occur after forbidding Evelyn to use her cell phone. [1] Asking Lucia to be explicit about her motives and expectations about banning Evelyn's cell phone use could create an opening to work with her and explain the downsides of this harsh punishment.

E. Work with Lucia to find a way of balancing her religious values with the necessity of all the family members respecting each other even when they have a disagreement. You could also say this balance is syntonic with the key religious values of respect, mercy, and compassion. [1] This approach can help decrease conflicts by helping Lucia understand that she doesn't have to choose between her LGBTQ+ child and her faith. There are some behaviors that are very compatible with Lucia's religious principles, such as talking with Evelyn respectfully, requiring that other family members demonstrate respect for Evelyn even when they disagree, and advocating for her daughter when others mistreat her.

F. Tell Lucia that sexual orientation might be fluid in many adolescents and that Lucia's behavior of harsh punishment could reinforce the outcome she is trying to prevent. [2] This approach could decrease Lucia's arousal and give you more time to work with Evelyn on her effective assertiveness, allowing you to develop a clear understanding of whether Evelyn is in a process of questioning or has already defined her sexual orientation. However, there are some risks inherent to this maneuver: Lucia might think you are manipulating her, and Evelyn might start wondering if you are really providing her with an affirmative mental health care environment.

6. With regard to the increase in suicidal thoughts reported by Evelyn, what should you do?

   A. Considering that Evelyn has expressed an increase in suicidal ideation and that a change in Lucia's stance will take some time, recommend that Evelyn be admitted to an inpatient psychiatric facility. [2] If you detect that it is not possible to decrease the intensity of Lucia's rejecting behavior and you are not able to work effectively with Evelyn on the crisis plan, a short hospitalization may give you some time to address these issues. However, hospitalizing Evelyn to effect a change in Lucia's response may set an unsustainable precedent that can interfere with Evelyn's recovery more than it aids it.

   B. Assess the danger of the situation, differentiating suicidal ideation from true suicidal intention. [1] This is an essential first step in deciding whether and how (i.e., under what level of care) you can treat Evelyn at this moment.

   C. Ask Evelyn whether this increase in suicidal ideation is related to experiences of rejection she felt regarding Lucia's reaction. [1] Understanding the significance of these interpersonal experiences as triggers is a big first step toward improving Evelyn's avoidance and management of the experiences. It moves her understanding of suicidal ideation away from reactions to unwanted feelings and instead toward reactions that have meaning in her internal life and outside situations.

   D. Ask Lucia and Evelyn to sign a written contract that Evelyn will not self-harm or kill herself and that Lucia will not demonstrate judgmental homophobic behaviors. [3] Contracting for safety is usually not effective with patients with BPD, whose states of mind (and risk) can change quickly and dramatically. Understanding what prompts Evelyn's pattern of suicidal tendencies is critical for safety planning and as an alliance-building intervention when done collaboratively with Evelyn.

   E. After talking about ways that you will work with Lucia to improve Evelyn's safety, discuss how Evelyn can help herself when she is in situations or emotional states that lead to self-harm or an increase in her suicidal ideation. [1] A problem-solving effort emphasizing agency to manage safety will be valuable. Evelyn might be resistant, and this then becomes the central consideration.

F. Explain to Lucia that punishment as a response to sexual orientation is correlated with suicide. Then say to Lucia that you want to
find a way to respect her family's religious values and at the same
time protect Evelyn's life, asking how she could help you to do so.
[1] This can be helpful in increasing Lucia's accountability for her
rejecting behaviors. These interpersonal events can provoke anger,
self-harm, and oscillation to more unreachable states where Evelyn
would be at greater risk for suicidal behavior. You can provide this
psychoeducation to Lucia in a very objective and nonjudgmental
atmosphere, where you join efforts to do your very best to foster
stability for Evelyn. You can point out how Lucia can facilitate self-
confidence and independence in supporting Evelyn's choices.

G. Prescribe quetiapine 25 mg daily to decrease the risk of suicidal behaviors. [2] This approach can decrease your own anxiety, but no
data in adolescent BPD support use of quetiapine to decrease the
risk of suicide. Prescribing quetiapine could take up precious time
in the session that you could invest in focusing on psychosocial interventions.

H. Access Evelyn's crisis plan again and work with her on skills that
could be added to it. [1] Reviewing the crisis plan and relevant skills
can add continuity to Evelyn's treatment, helping her apply techniques that have already worked for her. This engages Evelyn in
solving her emotional problems with your assistance as designed
by her prior to becoming suicidal. Involving her as an active par-
ticipant in managing crises is optimal.

I. Ask Evelyn if there is anyone in her family who is more supportive
about sexual orientation who could be included in her treatment
to help her. [1] Having the collaboration of a more supportive and
accepting family member can increase Evelyn's social safety network, providing a valuable resource she might access if things get
worse in her house.

J. Tell Lucia that you are very concerned that Evelyn is without her
cell phone: "Remaining without a cell phone could seriously jeopardize the execution of our crisis plan, which includes calling me
or other supports to help her. Let's find parameters for its use that
both of you can agree on right now." [1] This can increase Evelyn's
safety and help you show a collaborative way of making an agreement about Evelyn's phone use. This also helps Lucia refocus on
the priority of stabilizing the situation in terms of Evelyn's BPD
symptoms rather than controlling her sexuality.

7. Regarding your late arrival to this appointment, you should

A. Apologize for being late, recognize that Evelyn is right to be upset, and ask her forgiveness for what you did. Tell her that after causing her such pain, you are feeling guilty, and you feel the current session is a lost cause. Then reschedule a new appointment free of charge as soon as possible. [3] This seems an overly apologetic approach, which could in turn make it difficult for Evelyn to deal with her own feelings of shame if she makes a mistake in the future.

B. Apologize for being late, then use this event as an opportunity to explain how interpersonal hypersensitivity might have contributed to her intense emotional response toward you. [3] It is very important to connect some of Evelyn's emotional reactions to interpersonal hypersensitivity, but in this specific situation, it is important to be human and professional in acknowledging your failure to be on time.

C. Say you are sad and sorry for being late and that if you were in her shoes, you would feel irritated and upset. Ask Evelyn to describe what she is feeling at this moment and work with her to find the most effective way to handle this situation. [1] With this approach, you use self-disclosure to own your mistake as a corrective experience, acting as a role model for helping Evelyn deal more effectively when she makes a mistake.

D. Apologize for being late and explain with genuine emotion the pressing demands that caused you to be late for this session. [3] The session is Evelyn's therapy; self-disclosure must be done for the benefit of the patient, not the therapist. Giving detailed information about the reasons you were late when she did not ask burdens the patient with unnecessary information about you or might create a role reversal in which she feels that she must take care of your needs.

E. Tell Evelyn that you notice she is upset with you and that this is fair because you were late. However, considering that you are not usually late, she should demonstrate more empathy for you, just as you did when she was late for some appointments in the past. [3] Again, this behavior could be seen as a way to blame her for your own mistake. Pointing out Evelyn's past lateness is not advised because it would demonstrate that your forgiveness regarding her mistakes was not genuine. Instead of focusing on fairness about standards of timeliness, keep in mind she is upset because you are important to her, and she has cause to be upset.

Case Vignette 3: Undiagnosed BPD Detected in a Therapeutic Impasse (Alexia)

Chapters illustrated: Chapter 2 ("Overall Principles"), Chapter 3 ("Making the Diagnosis and Providing Psychoeducation"), Chapter 4 ("Getting Started"), and Chapter 5 ("Managing Suicidality and Nonsuicidal Self-Injury")

Lois W. Choi-Kain, M.D., M.Ed.

This clinical vignette depicts the case of Alexia, an adolescent in a lengthy psychiatric hospitalization without improvement in restrictive eating, suicidality, and head banging. It illustrates common impasses that can occur on inpatient units when unstable therapeutic alliances and staff splitting occur in the absence of an acknowledged BPD diagnosis. This case example demonstrates the way that diagnostic disclosure and psychoeducation can frame a reorientation to a treatment that is not working in order to diminish splits, reestablish alliances, and return responsibility to patients and their families for managing safety.

Alternative Responses at Decision Points

You are a new staff clinician on a child psychiatry unit and are assigned Alexia, a 14-year-old adolescent girl who was admitted to the inpatient unit 4 months ago for treatment of restrictive eating, self-harm, suicidal behaviors, and school nonattendance. This is her third hospitalization in the past year. During the course of this inpatient stay, Alexia has had periods of improved mood, decreased urges to self-harm, and participation on unit activities. However, every time discharge is prepared, Alexia stops eating and lightly bangs her head at night, frequently leading to one-to-one supervision, without which she cannot sleep. During the day, Alexia withdraws to her room and hides under her blankets. At times, she yells at staff who prompt her to get dressed or go to meals. Sometimes this involves verbal altercations; at other times staff withdraw and leave her alone. Over time, staff have become increasingly divided in their attitudes toward Alexia, with a few staff members readily going to her side when she is head banging and others showing obvious frustration and withholding support. Eventually, Alexia began sleeping only on nights when staff with whom she feels comfortable are on the unit, and she has stopped eating altogether.

When you first meet with the clinical team on the unit, tensions are high. Staff express frustrations about the difficulty discharging Alexia. They criticize each other for promoting Alexia's self-destructive behavior. You ask what her diagnoses are and are told she has reactive attachment disorder, major depressive disorder, social anxiety disorder, and other specified feeding or eating disorder. Because of the difficulty managing her care on the unit, Alexia has been sent temporarily to the autism unit downstairs, where staff use applied behavioral analysis to help Alexia get up in the morning, shower, follow a schedule, and eat. (**Decision point 1**)

1. In response to this introduction to Alexia's case and the state of conflict in the team, you

    A. Say little to contain tensions, tell the team Alexia appears to be a complex case and might be a chronic patient, and reassure them she is off the unit for now. Tell the nurse manager separately that the staff splitting is harmful and that the one-to-one observation cannot continue when Alexia returns.

    B. Tell the clinical team that Alexia has BPD and should start DBT treatment as soon as it is available.

    C. Observe that members of the team are expressing difficulties achieving their goals in Alexia's care and that there are different opinions about how to interact with her. Validate that head banging is a stressful management concern on a unit. Tell the team you want to learn more from them, the patient, and her family to evaluate what is working and what is not working. Let them know you want to better understand Alexia diagnostically in order to develop a focused plan of treatment.

    D. Evaluate Alexia's medication regimen and start naltrexone for self-harm.

You spend time reading Alexia's record and learn that she is an anxious but academically gifted teen who excels in school but struggles socially. Alexia gets moody and withdrawn and severely diminishes her food intake for a week at a time. She started to cut herself when she was 12 years old. Prior to her current hospital admission, Alexia stopped going to school, stopped eating, and screamed at her parents when they tried to intervene. After an altercation with her parents about going back to school, Alexia took 20 tablets of acetaminophen and cut her arms superficially on both sides. Alexia sought her parents' help immediately, and they brought her to the hospital. No serious medical problems occurred from the ingestion or cuts. At the time, Alexia explained she was desperate to disappear but was not intending to die. There are no other suicidal behaviors or suicide attempts in her history. You meet with Alexia on the autism unit. (**Decision point 2**)

2. In your initial meeting with Alexia, you should first

    A. Evaluate Alexia's suicidal and self-harming urges to determine her safety to return to the care of your team.

    B. Tell Alexia you are new to the team and are interested in understanding better what has happened during her hospital stay. Tell her you are interested in hearing what she thinks is going well and not so well and what she wants from treatment so that you can be most prepared to be her ally in the treatment process.

    C. Tell Alexia that from what you know about her, you think she has BPD and you can tell her all about it.

    D. Ask Alexia if she can start eating two meals a day in order to return to the child psychiatry unit.

Alexia comes to meet you wrapped in a fleece blanket. She avoids eye contact at first. When you ask her about what has happened in the hospital, Alexia looks at you briefly and tells you she is certain everyone hates her and wants to punish her. After you sympathize by saying that it can be painful and lonely when it feels as if others do not like you, Alexia nods her head and says this always happens to her. Alexia describes getting close to specific staff and feeling understood by them when they stick up for her and take extra time to make sure she is OK. She goes on to complain about others who are rule focused and seem cold and uncaring when she is overwhelmed with distress. When Alexia is stressed, especially in response to an interpersonal event, she stops eating, which she states helps her lessen her intense emotions. Before you leave, using the suggested wording to explain the DSM-5 criteria (see Table 3–2 in Chapter 3, "Making the Diagnosis and Providing Psychoeducation"), you review features of BPD as they relate to Alexia's significant fears of being abandoned, her feelings of emptiness and anger, and the many ups and downs in her relationships. You tell her you appreciate her thoughtfulness in talking about her problems, which are understandable to you. Using the script for explaining the BPD diagnosis (see Figure 3–2 in Chapter 3), you tell Alexia her problems are ones many others struggle with and that they are consistent with a diagnosis that explains the range of problems she has. You explain she has BPD, which can get better over time and can be treated. Alexia sighs in relief and says she has finally found a doctor who can understand her. You ask her if she would like to work on how to manage her interactions with staff because they seem to cause her a lot of stress and discouragement. Alexia looks at you anxiously and asks if you can help her. She asks you if you will be her doctor if she moves back to the child psychiatry unit. **(Decision point 3)**

3. You respond to Alexia's request to move back to the child psychiatry unit by

A. Telling her you want to work with her on sensitivity to relationships so that she can gain more skill in getting the responses she wants from people more predictably.
B. Informing her that she will work only with staff who stick to the rules because you believe in her ability to habituate to environments with fewer caregivers.
C. Answering that you want to work with her and think the treatment can work better with modifications that will involve your depending on her ability to learn from you and the team on the other unit. To start, you will want her to do homework and write down some goals she has for her work here that will help her work more consistently with you and your team.
D. Recommending that she stay on the autism unit because it is a fresh start for her.

You meet Alexia's parents, Bill and Karen. After many years of failed fertility treatments, they adopted Alexia from a European orphanage when she was 5 years old. Bill and Karen tried their best to provide a loving home, but Alexia's early emotional and behavioral difficulties overwhelmed them. Over time, they were unable to manage and resorted to giving her what she wanted as a way to motivate her or calm her down. At admission, Bill and Karen were relieved to get help and grateful to staff, but as the admission has been more prolonged, they have been angry, blaming, and demanding of staff when Alexia stops eating or bangs her head. They express frustration about the treatment not working and only causing Alexia to get worse. (**Decision point 4**)

4. In response to Bill and Karen's complaints about the treatment so far, you

A. Agree with their complaints and inform them you plan to rearrange staff shifts so Alexia can get the best care possible.
B. Agree that treatment is not working and tell them you all need to evaluate why. Share your impression that the treatment can be improved with a new diagnostic focus.
C. Inquire about BPD symptoms using DSM-5 and share the diagnostic disclosure script. Provide psychoeducation about the interpersonal hypersensitivity model and how it applies to Alexia's problems on the unit. Ask Bill and Karen how the model applies to their struggles at home.
D. Ask them about their problems with fertility and their experience of adoption.

You review the DSM-5 symptoms of BPD. Bill and Karen give you examples of how the criteria apply to Alexia's behavior, agreeing with you that this diagnosis may fit better than the reactive attachment disorder diagnosis because there are just as many moments of Alexia being receptive to their affections and care as there are of anger. Using the interpersonal hypersensitivity model, you ask them how their own behavior might follow the patterns of rescue, punitive hostility, or withdrawal, and they are relieved to hear your understanding of their tendencies. Bill and Karen share their worries that their difficulties with Alexia mean they are bad parents. You point out how the hospital team sometimes may get caught in the same dilemma, and staying engaged without being permissive, indulgent, and rescuing may help Alexia manage her emotional reactions without self-destructive behaviors over time.

You return to the team meeting and briefly inquire about the team members' views of what needs to happen next. Some staff say that the team should show more understanding of Alexia's difficulties, and others say she needs to be held to the same expectations as other patients. Team members are divided in their views on whether Alexia should come back to the unit. (**Decision point 5**)

5. In response to the staff's views, you reply by saying that

   A. Staff appear to be involved in splitting and should trade places, meaning those who have been focused on following unit expectations should be more reassuring and those who have been more reassuring should be more focused on unit expectations.

   B. Everyone appears to want Alexia to progress in treatment, and their separate responses make sense but do not work well in opposition to each other. You define your goal as an inpatient team is to help patients get well enough to step down to a lower level of care and return to life outside the hospital.

   C. Staff should arrange an extra meeting to process the experience of the failed treatment and their feelings about Alexia and her parents.

   D. You have talked to Alexia and her parents about your impressions that Alexia has BPD. Ask the team what they know about the diagnosis and how to treat it. Using the diagnosis and the interpersonal hypersensitivity model, explain that the responses staff have had toward Alexia are understandable but point to how the team might improve its consistency to stabilize her care.

You work with Alexia and the autism unit staff to develop goals on their unit for the week. In order for Alexia to return to the child psychiatry unit, which you tell Alexia you would really like to see happen, you will be required to show that she can take care of herself in terms of eating at mealtime and sleeping at night. Alexia is already improving in these areas on the autism unit, and she completes her homework outlining her goals, which include returning to school.

When Alexia returns to the child psychiatry unit, the staff work more consistently to listen to her expressions of difficulty with eating and being alone at night, providing validation while still recommending that follow through on self-care is in line with her goals. They refrain from staying too focused on soothing her or on pressuring her to follow through, emphasizing their support of her ability to choose. Alexia improves consistently, eating one or two meals daily and refraining from head banging for 2 weeks, when you begin discharge planning. As discharge approaches, Alexia begins to retreat and stays in bed under her blankets for a day, stating she wants to disappear. Bill and Karen become frustrated again, stating they don't believe treatment will ever work and now do not believe the BPD diagnosis. (**Decision point 6**)

6. As a next step, you should

   A. Speak to Bill and Karen about their reaction and let them know that change takes time. Validate their concerns while pointing back to the interpersonal hypersensitivity model to normalize Alexia's setback as expectable when increases in independence are approaching.
   B. Ask the staff to tell Alexia you will speak to her when she gets dressed and out of bed.
   C. Go to Alexia and ask her what has happened and how you might work together toward her goal of getting the responses she wants from others. Ask her to link her feelings about discharge to her current behaviors.
   D. Plan a family meeting and continue discharge planning.

Alexia spends 2 more weeks on the unit, unevenly progressing toward sleeping more stably without withdrawal to her bed. She shares fears of leaving the unit, especially feeling overwhelmed about the prospect of returning to school, where she had had so many prior difficulties. You clarify that she wants to disappear because of feeling overwhelmed but has no plans to attempt suicide. You ask Alexia and her family if they prefer that the team speak to school staff or if they would like guidance in doing so themselves. With appropriate consents to speak to the school counselor, the team case manager works with Alexia, her parents, and the school counselor to create a manageable plan to complete schoolwork and arranges for the school counselor to help Alexia manage her social difficulties. After obtaining Alexia and her parents' permission, you inform the school of the new diagnosis and the formulation of her problems in terms of interpersonal hypersensitivity. Alexia starts doing schoolwork and builds confidence in her ability to manage.

Alexia's wish to disappear is less intense. You remind her that progress takes time and her steps forward will be challenging but that you have confidence she can manage with the improvements she has made in getting the support she needs. She is able to discharge to home. After 3 weeks, Alexia is readmitted when she tells her parents she wants to overdose on a bottle of acetaminophen. (**Decision point 7**)

7. When you see Alexia on the unit, you should

   A. Welcome her with enthusiasm, telling her you are glad to see her.
   B. Reevaluate her medication regimen and consider what might be added.
   C. Ask her to write a chain analysis of how her self-harm urges developed and ask about any interpersonal events that may have contributed.
   D. Set up a family meeting to discuss what happened and to review the safety plan.

Alexia is discharged after a 3-day stay and begins treatment with a child psychiatry fellow who just completed GPM-A training. You see Alexia again after 3 months, when she returns to the unit with suicidal ideation and a plan to overdose on acetaminophen, which she has access to at home. The inpatient team engages in the same treatment plan, focusing on a chain analysis of events leading to hospitalization, discussion of what worked and did not work, and revision of the safety plan. Bill and Karen join a Family Connections group; they are calmer and therefore more able to listen to and validate Alexia.

Alexia talks openly about the painful interactions she has with peers and how they cause her to feel at times that everyone hates her. She now is able to independently recognize the sources of her suicidal urges and attempts to connect with friends or parents when she is feeling lonely or rejected. You remind her that these feelings will recur often, and her management of them can improve outcomes over time. With curiosity, you wonder out loud whether there is another way to manage than to be admitted. Alexia tells you that is exactly what her outpatient provider says to her and jokes he is more interested in her activities in clubs than in her symptoms. You comment that it sounds to you that they are both doing their jobs, which is a good outcome. Alexia is discharged after 3 days and does not return to the unit.

Discussion

1. In response to this introduction to Alexia's case and the state of conflict in the team, you

   A. Say little to contain tensions, tell the team Alexia appears to be a complex case and might be a chronic patient, and reassure them she is off the unit for now. Tell the nurse manager separately that the staff splitting is harmful and that the one-to-one observation cannot continue when Alexia returns. [3] Communication is essential in teams working with patients with complex difficulties such as Alexia. Saying very little while making changes in the availability of staff at night does not provide adequate explanation for why actions are being taken and will run the risk of aggravating both Alexia's symptoms and staff splitting. Although decreasing the reinforcing elements of the team's response to Alexia is warranted, doing so in a manner that involves both the staff as a team and the patient as a collaborator is preferred over unilateral action. There is not enough evidence that Alexia will be a chronic patient, and declaring her to be one will reduce hope.

B. Tell the clinical team that Alexia has BPD and should start DBT treatment as soon as it is available. [3] Although your intuition may be accurate, gathering more information to bring the patient, family, and team into a collaborative discussion about the BPD diagnosis provides the foundation of a thoughtful assessment and is optimal for building an alliance with all parties. Diagnostic disclosure in a context of frustration and tension can also undermine its validity when it is cast as an explanation for staff frustrations rather than a guiding point of the treatment plan. Starting with a framework that can educate, orient, and empower all involved is preferred as an initial step before involving specialists, who may ultimately be necessary. Alexia is returning to your care soon, and finding a way to solve the clinical problems that are immediately evident in inpatient management is the task at hand.

C. Observe that members of the team are expressing difficulties achieving their goals in Alexia's care and that there are different opinions about how to interact with her. Validate that head banging is a stressful management concern on a unit. Tell the team you want to learn more from them, the patient, and her family to evaluate what is working and what is not working. Let them know you want to better understand Alexia diagnostically in order to develop a focused plan of treatment. [1] When you start with shared observation, curiosity, and an interest in dialogue, it will be easier to build the teamwork necessary for Alexia's care. Sharing observations in the here and now enlists joint attention and can organize others in being on the same side instead of in a split. Being clear about your plan and open to others' views is a stance compatible with the GPM-A approach. Showing that you want to learn more about the case before making decisions also sets a tone of thinking first before acting. By pointing to the diagnostic assessment as an organizing structure for care, you can reorient the team to revising their responses. Last, speaking to the patient and family first before providing the diagnosis will allow them to be more involved as well so that their anticipation and investment in any changes to the treatment plan will make sense to them. This collaborative orientation is more likely to enlist their cooperation rather than to generate resistance.

D. Evaluate Alexia's medication regimen and start naltrexone for self-harm. [3] Reevaluating the medication regimen may be warranted, but evaluation of the diagnostic framework will help as a first step to a rational approach guided by evidence. No medication has been consistently shown to be effective for the treatment of self-harm (Hawton et al. 2015).

2. In your initial meeting with Alexia, you should first

A. Evaluate Alexia's suicidal and self-harming urges to determine her safety to return to the care of your team. [3] Although self-harming behaviors are certainly an appropriate concern in the clinical management of Alexia's care, putting those behaviors in context of life difficulties will help you and the patient make more sense of why those behaviors arise and what can be done instead. However, centering your treatment relationship in its first step on managing safety may interfere with building a dialogue about the larger context of Alexia's interpersonal hypersensitivity and the factors that cause suicidality and self-harm.

B. Tell Alexia you are new to the team and are interested in understanding better what has happened during her hospital stay. Tell her you are interested in hearing what she thinks is going well and not so well and what she wants from treatment so that you can be most prepared to be her ally in the treatment process. [1] Providing a focus and showing interest in what Alexia thinks and wants are important for setting the stage for you and Alexia to work collaboratively. Because Alexia is 14, this approach will likely be helpful because she is being treated as someone with her own motivations and perspective—a very important stance to take with adolescents. Knowing how Alexia sees her current situation, the problems in it, and what she wants from treatment will provide a basis for developing goals for which she can be motivated. Talking about her immediate situation also allows you to assess her self-awareness, her ability to understand social interactions, and what might be most important to her during the time she is in the hospital.

C. Tell Alexia that from what you know about her, you think she has BPD and you can tell her all about it. [3] Diving in immediately with your diagnostic impressions prior to allowing Alexia to share her point of view is a risky way to start. This way of taking over with what you know may put too much emphasis on your contribution to understanding and solving her problems. Trying to tell Alexia what is wrong with her on the basis of information from other people and without talking to her first is likely to turn her off and make her resistant to accepting the diagnosis. Skipping consideration of her unique point of view also misses an opportunity to have her contribute to building a shared perspective on her problems. It prevents her from being active in understanding her own problems, missing an opportunity of intervention in the sense that she is not thinking, but instead the clinician is the only one thinking.

D. Ask Alexia if she can start eating two meals a day in order to return to the child psychiatry unit. [3] This would be premature because you have not asked Alexia what she wants, including whether or not she wants to return to the unit or what is causing her to stop eating. Attempts to control behavior without understanding what is behind it may provide temporary solutions rather than longer-term resolution. Such attempts broker compliance rather than enlisting real collaboration. They also inadvertently model and reinforce the action-based approach to addressing Alexia's difficulties that has been failing her since before she was admitted.

3. You respond to Alexia's request to move back to the child psychiatry unit by

A. Telling her you want to work with her on sensitivity to relationships so that she can gain more skill in getting the responses she wants from people more predictably. [1] Alexia has a range of symptoms and will need a focus in order to work steadily on her problems on the unit and feel successful in taking steps forward. This focus also acknowledges the importance of other people's reactions to her, which she states is her main problem. Using the BPD diagnosis and the details Alexia herself shares about her difficulties on the unit, you can aim your joint attention at the clinical problem that needs to be solved for the case to move forward.

B. Informing her that she will work only with staff who stick to the rules because you believe in her ability to habituate to environments with fewer caregivers. [3] Although this is certainly the ultimate goal, you will need to work toward it with steps that are not as threatening to Alexia in terms of her connection to others, which can be used to help her be receptive to learning what she needs to complete her inpatient treatment. Making "you can do it" statements without acknowledgment of the related difficulties can result in withdrawal and fearful avoidance.

C. Answering that you want to work with her and think the treatment can work better with modifications that will involve your depending on her ability to learn from you and the team on the other unit. To start, you will want her to do homework and write down some goals she has for her work here that will help her work more consistently with you and your team. [1] You can accept Alexia's current idealization and proactively link your work to activity she does to change her situation. Setting the expectation that you will work together, and that she will need to stay active between interactions with you, particularly with staff, waters down the notion of an exclusive relationship with you. It also encourages a sense of agency in relation to her improvement and makes her more accountable.

D. Recommending that she stay on the autism unit for now because it is a fresh start for her. [2] The break from the unit can be used explicitly to reorganize the treatment plan and provide a fresh start. However, it will be important to confront what has been unfolding on the unit prior to Alexia's move because it reflects the very problems she encounters at home and also likely at school. Because she is now interested in returning to your unit, you can work with the team on the autism unit to set behavioral goals she can meet to be eligible for return. This makes the most of her time there and ties her behavior to the response she wants from you.

4. In response to Bill and Karen's complaints about the treatment so far, you

A. Agree with their complaints and inform them you plan to rearrange staff shifts so Alexia can get the best care possible. [3] This response would feed the splits that are interfering with the patient's use of treatment. It is important to validate Alexia's parents but to do so constructively in a way that allows integration of the team, and better understanding of Alexia's problems is preferred.

B. Agree that treatment is not working and tell them you all need to evaluate why. Share your impression that the treatment can be improved with a new diagnostic focus. [1] Setting the stage for diagnostic disclosure related to the parents' stated complaints will convey that they are heard and allows you to explain changes in the treatment approach.

C. Inquire about BPD symptoms using DSM-5 and share the diagnostic disclosure script. Provide psychoeducation about the interpersonal hypersensitivity model and how it applies to Alexia's problems on the unit. Ask Bill and Karen how the model applies to their struggles at home. [1] You can use the BPD diagnosis as an explanation for the interpersonal dynamics Alexia is facing on the unit to focus on a problem to be treated rather than a personalized complaint about specific staff. By relating these problems on the unit to the very problems Bill and Karen have also faced allows you to validate their difficulties managing the special needs Alexia has in her care while also facilitating a more sympathetic view of the staff. You can provide Bill and Karen information about BPD, starting with the BPD Brief and Family Guidelines (Gunderson and Berkowitz 2006a; 2006b) (see Appendix D).

D. Ask them about their problems with fertility and their experience of adoption. [3] Although their history of becoming parents will be relevant to understanding their dynamics with Alexia, sticking with a here and now focus on the immediate clinical problems on the unit provides more clear avenues to teamwork and resolution of the current difficulties in the treatment. Work related to Bill and Karen's history as parents can be reserved for the outpatient phase once Alexia is discharged.

5. In response to the staff's views, you reply by saying that

A. Staff appear to be involved in splitting and should trade places, meaning those who have been focused on following unit expectations should be more reassuring and those who have been more reassuring should be more focused on unit expectations. [3] Splitting is a useful concept to explain the division in the staff, but in and of itself it does not point to a coherent treatment plan. It may be a good idea for staff to balance their responses to Alexia, but simply trading places may not be sufficient for them to understand her problems in a way that generates more teamwork. This intervention would perpetuate a split in the team and in Alexia's experience on the unit.

B. Everyone appears to want Alexia to progress in treatment, and their separate responses make sense but do not work well in opposition to each other. You define your goal as an inpatient team is to help patients get well enough to step down to a lower level of care and return to life outside the hospital. [1] This statement joins the team's views and validates both sides. Reuniting those sides according to a shared goal that defines the role of the inpatient team can organize team dynamics in the context of Alexia's care.

C. Staff should arrange an extra meeting to process the experience of the failed treatment and their feelings about Alexia and her parents. [3] It is important to acknowledge the strong feelings staff may have about the difficulties of Alexia's care. However, prioritizing an unstructured conversation about their emotional reactions rather than the treatment plan moving forward may keep the focus on emotional reactions rather than a clinical understanding of Alexia's psychiatric problems.

D. You have talked to Alexia and her parents about your impressions that Alexia has BPD. Ask the team what they know about the diagnosis and how to treat it. Using the diagnosis and the interpersonal hypersensitivity model, explain that the responses staff have had toward Alexia are understandable but point to how the team might improve its consistency to stabilize her care. [1] This response allows you to share your thinking with the team while also incorporating both sides' views of what needs to be done. It also educates staff, who may not know much about BPD. Staff may bring up myths and misinformation about BPD that you can dispel by using information on the myths of BPD (see Table 1 in the Preface) and top 10 reasons for early intervention for BPD (see Table 2 in the Preface).

6. As a next step, you should

A. Speak to Bill and Karen about their reaction and let them know that change takes time. Validate their concerns while pointing back to the interpersonal hypersensitivity model to normalize Alexia's setback as expectable when increases in independence are approaching. [1] Being nonreactive to these expectable developments and remaining supportive and engaged when the patient or family is angry will allow you to convey your ongoing availability in Alexia's care. You can understand their fears of symptomatic behaviors and their anticipated inability to handle them at home.

Emphasize their need for support and point them to resources such as Family Connections (see "National Education Alliance for Borderline Personality Disorder (NEABPD)" in Appendix E, "Online Psychoeducation Resources"), which can provide ongoing psychoeducation and support from other families going through the same experience (Hoffman et al. 2005).

B. Ask the staff to tell Alexia you will speak to her when she gets dressed and out of bed. [3] Knowing that Alexia might be fearful of abandonment as she approaches discharge, conveying your unavailability runs the risk of aggravating her withdrawal and may result in a continued path to returning to the prior treatment impasse.

C. Go to Alexia and ask her what has happened and how you might work together toward her goal of getting the responses she wants from others. Ask her to link her feelings about discharge to her current behaviors. [1] Returning to shared goals allows a platform of joining the patient without necessarily reinforcing her avoidance. Alexia is likely not yet aware of the connection between her regression and her fear of being discharged. Your response provides a focus for how you and Alexia can work together and allows her to provide input on a solution to the current stressor of discharge. This may allow her to acknowledge her fears of leaving.

D. Plan a family meeting and continue discharge planning. [1] Increasing sources of support that will remain available after Alexia leaves will be necessary to prepare her parents for the challenges ahead. Anticipate difficulties and provide proactive guidance about how Bill and Karen might respond so that they are able to remain available and involved in a way that allows Alexia to make choices.

7. When you see Alexia on the unit, you should

A. Welcome her with enthusiasm, telling her you are glad to see her. [3] Noticing that Alexia was able to ask for help without self-harming is important. It is also important to note to Alexia that being able to manage these moments without disrupting her engagement in other aspects of her life is the best way to promote recovery from BPD and rehabilitation from her lengthy hospital stay.

B. Reevaluate her medication regimen and consider what might be added. [3] There is no evidence that medication changes would be helpful at this juncture. Recurrence of urges to self-harm as a patient faces usual stressors outside the hospital is expected, and because no medication is proven to consistently improve self-harm, starting medication changes is not recommended. Additionally, medication changes can problematically focus solutions on what clinicians can provide rather than on what patients and their families can do to manage outside the hospital.

C. Ask her to write a chain analysis of how her self-harm urges developed and ask about any interpersonal events that may have contributed. [1] Involving Alexia in understanding what factors lead to hospitalization allows her to continue to build agency and involvement in solving her own problems. Building her confidence to be able to do so, even in the course of setbacks, is desirable. A sample chain analysis is provided in Figure 4–2 in Chapter 4, "Getting Started."

D. Set up a family meeting to discuss what happened and to review the safety plan. [1] The family will need help as well to know what they can do to support Alexia when she has urges to hurt herself. Reviewing the plan and reminding the patient and her family what they can do in moments of self-harm urges can refocus their efforts on refining what they do outside the hospital rather than needing to return to establish safety. This will take some steps after a lengthy hospitalization. Psychoeducation about how building a life outside the hospital provides opportunities for building self-esteem and relationships that can buffer Alexia's vulnerabilities will redirect the family to the opportunity for recovery outside the hospital.

Case Vignette 4: Pharmacotherapy and GPM for Adolescents With BPD (Maddie)

Chapters illustrated: Chapter 4 ("Getting Started") and Chapter 6 ("Pharmacotherapy and Comorbidity")

Carl Fleisher, M.D.

This case illustrates key principles of applying the GPM model to treat adolescents with BPD and the role, limits, and management of medication as an adjunct to case management. As with all interventions in GPM, treatment should employ medications that work. Those that do not work should be stopped.

GPM for adolescents encourages providers to initiate discussion proactively about issues specific to this stage of development. Two such issues pertain to the effects of medication: the FDA black box warning for SSRIs and weight gain from antipsychotic medication. The latter may be addressed in the wider context of nutrition and overall adolescent health. There are three other issues addressed in this vignette that are specific to adolescence: social media use (in the broader context of negotiating between adolescents' drive for independence and parents' desire to supervise and protect their children), collaboration with schools, and sexual health.

GPM-A encourages providers to avoid prescribing medication but acknowledges the reality that many patients still receive it for one reason or another. When medication is considered, providers play a crucial role in setting patients' and families' expectations. This includes discussing potential harms, explaining monitoring requirements, and emphasizing caution about attributing benefit or harm to medication (whether during use or discontinuation). When medication is prescribed, we recommend that providers orient patients and families to attend to specific goals and effects rather than to the presence or absence of unwanted thoughts or feelings. Setting goals for medication also helps limit its duration of use. Alternatively, providers can recommend using medication only for a prespecified amount of time. Overall, when it comes to prescribing for adolescents, GPM espouses patience, healthy reluctance, and thoughtful use of nonmedical supports and collaboration.

Alternative Responses at Decision Points

Choose 1=helpful; 2=possibly helpful, with continuing reservations; 3=not helpful—or even harmful

> Maddie, a 16-year-old girl, is brought by her parents to see you to establish outpatient care after stepping down from a residential treatment program. She was referred to residential treatment because depression and frequent mood changes prevented her from attending school with any regularity.
>
> At the treatment program, Maddie was diagnosed with BPD. The diagnosis was based on a history of impairment stemming from her clinging frantically to relationships. She partied and did drugs because that was what her friends were doing; she welcomed flirtation from boys and quickly formed intense relationships with them. She did not express any needs of her own, lest the other person leave the relationship, to the point where she didn't know really who she was. She tended to remain submissive and put others on a pedestal, ignoring clearly undesirable qualities— until someone new expressed interest in connecting with her. Then, her

opinion of current relationship partners would flip, and she suddenly felt disgusted by them. Her moods shifted constantly, depending wholly on the currents of these bumpy relationships. She rapidly felt worse, for example, if a friend or partner did not respond to a text message or if she saw posts on social media showing that friends had gathered without her. These perceived slights made Maddie feel worthless and unlovable, and her reactions were so strong that her only tool to escape the pain was to scratch or cut herself repeatedly. Once she had self-harmed "enough," her emotions seemed to vanish, leaving her feeling comfortably numb. If she did not have the means to self-harm, her emotions would intensify until the world around her did not feel real.

Maddie was also diagnosed with major depressive disorder, in partial remission, and had a history of bulimia nervosa. Two weeks into residential treatment, a psychiatrist prescribed an SSRI for her depression, titrated to the maximum FDA-approved dose. Maddie was discharged 2 weeks after that, when her mood stabilized enough to allow her to start catching up on schoolwork.

You review the diagnosis of BPD first with Maddie alone, then with her parents. You provide psychoeducation about the interpersonal hypersensitivity model, explaining, "We all need relationships and feel hurt after a rejection, but for some people rejection would feel so terrible that they'll do almost anything to avoid it." You then review the course and treatment of BPD. Maddie's parents express dismay, saying that they searched extensively but could not find any affordable providers in the area who offer DBT. You respond with sympathy, noting that although you are not an expert, you do have training in GPM-A for BPD. You express confidence that Maddie's life can improve through her participation in therapy that focuses on achieving concrete goals, supporting academic achievement, and monitoring progress—with or without episodic use of medication. The family is encouraged by the hope you convey, and they agree to engage in weekly treatment.

In your office, you note that Maddie is dressed in stylishly ripped jeans and a hoodie. She says she feels "fine," and when you ask her to elaborate, she says "Just fine, like in the middle." She is sleeping 6–7 hours a night. She reports no side effects from her medication. Her parents, however, are concerned because she has attended school only 50% of the time in the 2 weeks that she has been home.

Maddie's mother adds that she has been monitoring Maddie's activity on social media, when Maddie suddenly interrupts, saying angrily, "You don't know what you're talking about, Mom! Those are my friends, and you can't just go snooping around to read what we talk about!" Maddie's mother continues talking to you, sharing her observation that Maddie seems overly sensitive to her friends' comments. Maddie again interrupts, in a raised voice, saying, "What are you talking about? I'm not sensitive, Mom. You're just dumb and you don't get it. Doc, just ignore her; everything with my friends is fine!" Wanting to build rapport, you respond in an understanding tone, "Sure, sure, OK, Maddie." She calms visibly on hearing that, so you ask her what her mother is so concerned about if everything with friends is going well. Maddie throws up her arms as she replies, "I have no idea! She's always suspicious of what I do. Honestly, I think she just doesn't understand how teenagers talk to each other."

Regarding her recent absences from school, Maddie explains that she has felt overwhelmed by the full load of school assignments. On top of that, she admits her moods can still get intense if she feels criticized by peers in her classroom. She is upset that her parents don't give her privacy and don't have any confidence in her capacity to handle her current situation. She insists that her overall ability to cope in school is improving. Noting this disagreement, you encourage Maddie to set a goal of convincing her parents to express more confidence and stop monitoring her social media accounts. Maddie's parents, in contrast, ask to set a treatment goal of her getting back on track with adolescent development. They want her to attend school 100% of the time and join an after-school activity. If she does both of those things, they are willing to pull back from monitoring her social media use.

Maddie's parents, worrying that she will spiral back into avoiding school, ask you whether her medication should be changed, whether they should take away her phone, and how to get her to attend school consistently. (**Decision points 1–3**)

1. What might be an appropriate recommendation regarding Maddie's medication?

    A. No change.
    B. Titrate the current SSRI. Maddie may experience greater improvement even at doses above FDA-approved maximum.
    C. Change to an alternative SSRI.
    D. Add a mood stabilizer.
    E. Add a second-generation antipsychotic.

2. How would you recommend Maddie's family support the appropriate use of social media?

    A. Maddie should delete her accounts and apps, and her parents should take away her phone for a month.
    B. One of Maddie's parents should read everything Maddie is planning to post to make sure it is appropriate.
    C. Maddie and her parents can meet on their own time to discuss various options and make a compromise about what type and degree of supervision they are comfortable with.
    D. Maddie needs to agree to give her parents the passwords to her social media accounts so they can monitor all of her activity.
    E. Maddie's parents can allow her a small amount of time each day to use social media at home to try to keep her from getting too engrossed or too upset.

3. What is the best way to address Maddie's difficulty attending school?

   A. Maddie and her parents should seriously consider an internet-based homeschool program.

   B. One of Maddie's parents should offer to drive her to school every morning to make sure she gets there.

   C. You should call the school to recommend that Maddie be allowed to turn assignments in late.

   D. You should call the school to recommend that they reduce Maddie's classwork and homework for 2 weeks.

   E. Maddie's parents should send her to boarding school, where she cannot run away from her problems.

On the basis of the first meeting with Maddie, you consider watching and waiting but ultimately recommend a new antidepressant trial because Maddie is having such difficulty with school reentry, ongoing mood symptoms, and conflict with her parents about how to proceed. You encourage the family to discuss together how Maddie can manage her presence on social media with an appropriate level of supervision, offering some tips from what other families have told you worked for them. You also ask her parents to contact the school counselor to see whether it would be appropriate to lighten her workload temporarily. You inform her parents that you can make yourself available to school staff if they want your input.

You review the risks, benefits, side effects, and alternatives of a new SSRI. When discussing side effects, you make sure to mention both the FDA black box warning about suicidal ideation and the fact that there is very little research in adolescents regarding medications for BPD. Maddie and her parents had not heard this information before; they are surprised. They appreciate your detailed discussion of how to put the black box warning in context, allowing them to trust in what you think would be the best step going forward. You recommend a cross-taper from the current SSRI to the new one, rather than discontinuing the current medication first, in the hopes of hastening an improvement in function. You make it clear that medication is viewed as a temporary intervention, requiring measurable goals to be able to assess how long to continue its use. Together with Maddie and her parents, you decide on a goal of 80% school attendance and/or a return to baseline academic performance (Bs). You also offer to call the school administration, knowing that you can refer them to helpful resources such as Project Air or DBT in Schools.

Two weeks later, however, in the midst of the cross-taper, Maddie returns to your office with her parents. She is unhappy that, since starting the new SSRI, her jaw aches on awakening. Her experience of her emotions is also much diminished, including happiness, but she says she doesn't mind this nearly as much as her jaw pain. Her school attendance is now above 90%. Her parents ask you whether the medication caused her pain and, if so, what you suggest they do. (**Decision point 4**)

4. What might be an appropriate recommendation for Maddie's medication?

A. No change.

B. Switch to a second-generation antipsychotic.

C. Discontinue medications while asking Maddie to continue to monitor her response.

D. Reverse course: discontinue the newer SSRI and continue treatment with the original one.

E. Switch to a mood stabilizer.

In an effort to manage the medication conservatively, you opt to discontinue the newer SSRI and continue the current dose of the original one, which was well tolerated at least. Maddie's jaw pain subsides rapidly, and her moods are no longer blunted. Over the subsequent month, she attends school consistently. She sleeps 7 hours a night, her grades rise, and she joins the school volleyball team. Then, in a follow-up session, Maddie is pleased to tell you that she has a new boyfriend, someone she met while in the residential treatment program. They had been exchanging text messages and, because he lives in the same area, gradually started spending time together. You make sure to ask her about safe sexual practices. She feels criticized by the question, so you explain that you discuss this topic routinely with all teenage patients and that you hope she does not take it personally.

After 2 months of uneventful weekly sessions, Maddie's mother contacts you to let you know that her daughter overdosed on the SSRI and is being admitted to a nearby psychiatric hospital. She describes Maddie as despondent that her boyfriend did not show up for a planned date after not responding to any of her communications for 3 days. Immediately prior to hospitalization, Maddie had stopped doing homework. She was spending 2–3 hours trying to fall asleep. She cut herself to express how worthless and hopeless she felt; her parents saw the new cuts but chalked them up to stress from school. Maddie had not reached out to her friends for support because she assumed they were angry that she had been spending every day over the past few weeks with her boyfriend.

During admission, Maddie's SSRI is discontinued and lamotrigine is prescribed in its place. Quetiapine is added to address her insomnia. Her thoughts of suicide wane in the first few days of the hospitalization, only to return as her inpatient providers begin to discuss discharge. They increase her dose of lamotrigine and ultimately discharge her 10 days after admission.

In her first session after discharge, Maddie reports that she feels "good." She says she appreciates how she overreacted to her (now ex-) boyfriend being out of contact. She thinks the medicine must be helping her feel better. She is sleepy at night but not groggy in the morning. She looks forward to returning to school and catching up on work she missed. You alert her and her parents to the need for periodic laboratory tests while she is taking quetiapine. They agree to testing but ask if it is necessary for her to keep taking this medication. You were going to ask them the same question, so you engage them in discussion. During this discussion, you also aim to address the hospitalization. (**Decision points 5 and 6**)

5. What, if any, changes would you make in Maddie's medication regimen?

    A. Add low-dose lithium to target her recent suicidality.
    B. Discontinue quetiapine. She was sleeping fine prior to hospitalization, so it is unlikely she will need it for long in the outpatient setting.
    C. Discontinue quetiapine. Patients should not be prescribed antipsychotics to treat insomnia.
    D. No change, with a goal to continue this regimen.
    E. No change, with a goal to discontinue one or both medications eventually.

6. What issue(s) regarding Maddie's hospitalization do you want to be sure to address?

    A. Encourage a targeted family discussion about specific actions Maddie's parents can take to support her when she feels overwhelmed or suicidal.
    B. Make a verbal or written agreement that she will contact you first if in the future she again feels the desire to overdose.
    C. Look back with Maddie at the events leading up to her overdose to find opportunities where she could have coped in other ways.
    D. Be sure Maddie acknowledges that hospitalization only encourages regression; she should make better use of her crisis plan.
    E. Reflect with Maddie and her parents about whether her hospitalization indicates that the current treatment is not effective and should stop.

For the moment, you opt to leave Maddie's medications as they are, but you aim to try discontinuing them at a point when her function is more stable. Two months later, Maddie returns to your office just for a medication management visit. She has continued to attend school and is keeping up with homework. She was voted co-captain of her volleyball team. Her moods have been good overall. She sleeps well, and her peer relationships are relatively stable. Additionally, you mention that the results of her fasting bloodwork were all normal. She is pleased but notes that her appetite has increased significantly. When she stands on the scale, you and she realize that she has gained 10 pounds since the last visit (about 7% of her body weight). She is upset about the weight gain and asks you what can be done. (**Decision point 7**)

7. How would you manage Maddie's medication regimen in light of this new complication?

   A. Prescribe appetite-suppressing medication such as luraglutide to counteract appetite increase from quetiapine.

   B. No change: some people gain weight while taking antipsychotics, but 7% of body weight is not much and she may not gain any more.

   C. Discontinue quetiapine and check in after 2 weeks to see how she is doing.

   D. Offer her and her parents psychoeducation about weight gain (e.g., managing caloric intake, portion control, purchasing healthy foods, limiting snacks).

   E. Discontinue quetiapine and replace it with clonidine to be sure insomnia does not return.

Maddie and her parents are too nervous about insomnia reemerging to discontinue quetiapine, despite the weight gain, so you agree to continue it for a short while longer. Your agreement stipulates that any further weight gain would automatically be cause for discontinuation. Two weeks later, although Maddie has made efforts to reduce her caloric intake, she has gained another 3 pounds. Thus, you discontinue quetiapine.

Over the next 9 months, Maddie regularly attends both school and therapy with you. In one session, she grows unusually quiet, and you ask her if something is going on. She says there is but wants you to promise you won't tell her parents anything before she tells you more. You reemphasize the commitment you made when treatment started to protect her right to privacy in the absence of any immediate threat. Reassured, she describes that she has been eating more recently because she came across a reminder of something that happened when she was 12 that made her feel very ashamed. You express empathy and ask whether she is in any current danger; she is not. You invite her to say more. She does not want to ruin her own good mood, so she tells you she will talk about it another time.

Also over these months, several challenges arise in Maddie's life: She starts dating a new boy, but he breaks up with her. Her friend group shifts as she drifts away from peers she met in treatment programs. Her brother goes to college, leaving her the only child at home with her parents. In sessions, you listen as she describes her difficulties. You encourage her to identify her feelings, then use that awareness to make informed choices about relationships. You also encourage her to connect with new peers through after-school activities. There, she can make friends because of common interests rather than common illness or to counter abandonment fears. During these stressful situations, Maddie uses coping skills from the crisis plan you created with her and even starts to open up more to her parents.

Maddie, by now 17 years old, demonstrates an increasing ability to regulate her emotions appropriately and effectively. In light of that fact, she would like to discontinue the lamotrigine. However, her parents dislike that idea. They fear suicidality will quickly return, and they expect her to need medication for many years anyway because of her diagnosis. The three of them turn to you; all seem to expect you will agree with her parents. (**Decision point 8**)

8. Would you make any changes to Maddie's medication regimen at this point?

   A. No change: she has not had stable function long enough to justify that.
   B. Taper and discontinue lamotrigine. You expect this will destabilize Maddie emotionally, but you hope it will help her trust that you are listening to her needs.
   C. No change: although Maddie is functioning well, she can continue to take lamotrigine safely for a long time.
   D. Taper and discontinue lamotrigine; no evidence supports long-term medication use, plus Maddie has demonstrated a meaningful period of emotional resilience.
   E. Switch to an SSRI because SSRIs are safe for long-term use and you can avoid even a remote risk of Maddie developing Stevens-Johnson syndrome.

Discussion

1. What might be an appropriate recommendation regarding Maddie's medication?

   A. No change. [2] Maddie is struggling to attend school 2 weeks after stepping down from a higher level of care. This problem often generates a sense of urgency in providers, parents, or both to "do something" that will improve attendance. Taking their concerns seriously can help build the alliance.
   B. Titrate the current SSRI. Maddie may experience greater improvement even at doses above FDA-approved maximum. [3] There is no research in adolescents to support titrating SSRIs beyond the FDA-approved maximum doses to treat symptoms of BPD or depression.
   C. Change to an alternative SSRI. [2] This is a tempting choice because it is a concrete action in a situation where the patient's impairment creates a strong urge to "do something." Because there are other indications that the patient is not coping well (e.g., lability, sensitivity), switching to an alternative SSRI might be justified. On the other hand, a change in medication may not impact Maddie's

school attendance. Listening to her explanation for skipping school may uncover opportunities to offer other interventions to improve her attendance.

D. Add a mood stabilizer. [3] The GPM model recommends against polypharmacy. There are no indications that a mood stabilizer is needed. If the first medication is not adequately effective, then the GPM model would recommend discontinuing it before trying any other medication.

E. Add a second-generation antipsychotic. [3] The GPM model recommends against polypharmacy. There are no indications that an antipsychotic is needed. If the first medication is not adequately effective, then the GPM model would recommend it be discontinued before trying any other medication.

Principles and clinical pearls for decision point 1:

- There is no research to suggest that prescribing doses of any medication above the FDA-approved maximum will provide additional benefit to patients with BPD.
- The GPM model stresses avoiding medication use, especially polypharmacy, whenever possible. Seemingly dire situations may fade with the passage of time or be overtaken by a new crisis that grips everyone's attention.
- If patients tell you they feel overwhelmed, it is important to recognize that such feelings are common in the process of stepping down from a higher level of care. In GPM-A, the clinician is encouraged to collaborate with the patient, parents, school (and therapist, in split treatments) to address psychosocial needs and challenges; making these the primary targets of intervention will hopefully address feeling overwhelmed and obviate any desire for medication.

2. How would you recommend Maddie's family support the appropriate use of social media?

A. Maddie should delete her accounts and apps, and her parents should take away her phone for a month. [3] Parents often have an understandable reflex to take away anything that is used inappropriately. However, removing access to social contact will generally be experienced as harsh by adolescents and thus hinder their relationship with their parents. Regardless of how it is perceived, this punishment also will not fix Maddie's problem of poor judgment under stress.

B. One of Maddie's parents should read everything Maddie is planning to post to make sure it is appropriate. [2] This approach could work in the short run, but it is impractical for parents, will be experienced by adolescents as highly intrusive, and worst of all, will reduce agency. Instead, it might be effective to incorporate this as one option or strategy within a broader plan to teach and strengthen Maddie's own responsible social media use.

C. Maddie and her parents can meet on their own time to discuss various options and make a compromise about what type and degree of supervision they are comfortable with. [1] As an expert, you can offer suggestions of what has worked for other families, you can shape the family's expectations about what is developmentally appropriate, and you can advocate for Maddie's needs in order to balance conversations that often devolve into power struggles.

D. Maddie needs to agree to give her parents the passwords to her social media accounts so they can monitor all of her activity. [2] This approach should be standard for tweens and early adolescents but may be inappropriate and feel intrusive to an older child like Maddie. There may be ways to achieve the same goal that are more collaborative and more nuanced (and less time intensive for her parents).

E. Maddie's parents can allow her a small amount of time each day to use social media at home to try to keep her from getting too engrossed or too upset. [2] This strategy tries to achieve the desired outcome in a neutral fashion by restricting the time to use social media rather than intervening in how Maddie engages. Such a strategy may not do much to strengthen her skills but nevertheless may be more palatable to Maddie because it does not pathologize or infantilize her.

Principles and clinical pearls for decision point 2:

- Adolescents' social media use is a thorny issue at the intersection of numerous psychological challenges: emotion regulation, impulse control, desires for independence, self-esteem, risk-taking, identity, peer attachment and connection, sexuality, bullying, and group dynamics, not to mention issues of information privacy, managing screen time, and the permanence of everything posted to the internet. We encourage the reader to appreciate that this complexity means all attempts to ensure appropriate social media engagement will have both drawbacks and advantages.

- Adolescents want to be able to engage on social media platforms skillfully in order to strengthen their relationships, raise their social standing, or boost their self-esteem. Any intervention that addresses social media use will ideally be geared toward teaching adolescents the knowledge and techniques they need to navigate the digital social world with confidence.
- Different frames of reference often reveal new opportunities to solve problems. Maladaptive social media use often occurs when adolescents spend inordinate amounts of time alone with their smartphones or when they feel lonely or are having trouble sleeping. Interventions that address those problems may indirectly improve social media use without requiring parents to resort to drastic or labor-intensive measures.

3. What is the best way to address Maddie's difficulty attending school?

   A. Maddie and her parents should seriously consider an internet-based homeschool program. [2] Homeschool programs come in various stripes and can be useful in bridging a return to a classroom setting. The danger to be wary of is that homeschool programs become a way to avoid social or educational challenges that should and can be surmounted. Used for avoidance, homeschooling could reduce agency and even paint Maddie as "too fragile" for a typical educational setting.

   B. One of Maddie's parents should offer to drive her to school every morning to make sure she gets there. [3] This tangible action may seem tempting in its (over)simplicity. In addition, shifting the responsibility of attendance toward the parents may reduce any sense of helplessness they feel. However, giving Maddie's parents more responsibility can undermine her sense of agency. Ultimately, this strategy does not address the reasons she avoids school. Likewise, it neither strengthens Maddie's capacities nor provides meaningful respite for her to strengthen her capacities by other means.

   C. You should call the school to recommend that Maddie be allowed to turn assignments in late. [2] Leniency on late assignments may indeed be a helpful component of a gradual, supported return to school following intensive treatment. This probably would not be sufficient, however.

   D. You should call the school to recommend that they reduce Maddie's classwork and homework for 2 weeks. [1] Assignments pile up quickly while adolescents attend treatment programs. The larger the stack of work to be done, the more discouraged an adolescent may become. Allowing a reduced workload is likely to lessen any trepidation Maddie might feel about getting back into the school routine. This, too, may not be wholly sufficient.

E. Maddie's parents should send her to boarding school, where she cannot run away from her problems. [3] Parents are commonly, and understandably, exasperated by the behavior of their children with a personality disorder. The idea of boarding (or military) school typically comes up when parents or providers imagine that all possible interventions with local resources have already failed. Sending Maddie away may relieve her parents of their distress but likely will not solve the problem. Adolescents often do poorly in school because of *how* interventions have been implemented, not because they were the wrong solutions. Moreover, adolescents with personality disorders who enroll in boarding school will continue to have symptoms in that setting yet lack ready access to clinical care. Adolescents may even view separation from family (at times correctly?) as an abandonment—a major blow for adolescents who are hypersensitive to rejection.

Principles and clinical pearls for decision point 3:

- Adolescents with personality disorders can thrive in a traditional classroom environment when properly supported, sometimes despite significant emotional turmoil. In addition, traditional schools and classrooms offer opportunities for social development that homeschool programs typically do not replicate. Hence, a return to a classroom environment should be the goal unless repeated attempts at reintegration have failed.
- It can be quite difficult for adolescents to reintegrate effectively into a traditional classroom environment. As with therapy, progress should be expected, and any support that might advance that progress should be considered. School staff need and typically wish for guidance in dealing with adolescents with a personality disorder. Even a 5-minute conversation with a teacher or counselor can greatly improve a school team's willingness to support these patients' needs. Providers who are pressed for time may rely on parents to educate school staff, or at least point them to useful internet-based resources (e.g., Project Air).
- Some schools do not provide academic accommodations to students with personality disorders because their grades are good. However, students like Maddie whose illness is sufficiently severe that they have attended residential treatment are deserving of at least the option to receive extra support. Patients' parents often need to be taught that

public schools are mandated by federal law to evaluate a student's need for extra support—but only if the request to do so is received in writing. More information about accommodations can be found at https://kidshealth.org/en/parents/iep.html.

4. What might be an appropriate recommendation for Maddie's medication?

   A. No change. [3] Maddie says she cannot tolerate the adverse effect she experiences, so it would be harmful, or at the least ineffective, to tell her to continue taking the medication.

   B. Switch to a second-generation antipsychotic. [3] Switching to another class of medication lacks a clear justification in the face of both improving function and a negligible history of medication trials.

   C. Discontinue medications while asking Maddie to continue to monitor her response. [1] GPM-A favors avoiding medication use whenever possible, so there is an even stronger justification to discontinue medication when it causes adverse effects. Discontinuing medication will often reveal that the patient functions equally well (or poorly) without medication as with it.

   D. Reverse course: discontinue the newer SSRI and continue treatment with the original one. [2] Because Maddie seemed to tolerate the original SSRI, it may be reasonable to prescribe that one (for now), especially because her school attendance is greatly improved.

   E. Switch to a mood stabilizer. [3] Switching to another class of medication lacks a clear justification in the face of both improving function and a negligible history of medication trials.

Principles and clinical pearls for decision point 4:

- There can be intense pressure to prescribe medication to adolescents who are functioning poorly—from parents, from the patient, from the larger health care organization, or from a therapist or another physician. One aspect of good care that can assist in resisting that pressure is to carefully explain the lack of justification for prescribing and the potentially serious risk involved. This generally works better when coupled with offering alternative solutions such as increasing the "dose" of therapy, adding a group therapy, or emphasizing the therapeutic value of greater involvement in after-school or weekend activities.

- It is hard to justify medication use in treating adolescent patients with BPD and even harder when medications cause adverse effects. Medications that do not provide a clear and compelling benefit—easily discerned when specific, collaborative goals have been formulated—should be discontinued (gradually, of course). Patients can be supported in managing their emotions by other means.

- Psychoeducation is a key component of the treatment of BPD; it plays many roles, especially when dealing with adolescents and their families (Flynn et al. 2017; Zanarini et al. 2018). Psychoeducation can help adolescents manage symptoms; it can help schools support students and lessen any worries their staff might have about patient safety; and it can ground parents in appropriate expectations regarding the effects of medication. Another potential benefit of psychoeducation could be that, in providing patients and their families with a sense of shared information or experience, families learn from observing a model for communicating more effectively.

5. What, if any, changes would you make in Maddie's medication regimen?

A. Add low-dose lithium to target her recent suicidality. [3] Lithium has been shown in research to reduce suicidality in adults with major depression, but that literature is not necessarily generalizable to adolescents with BPD. Suicidality in BPD can be understood differently from suicidality in major depression; generally speaking, it is transient and precipitated by real or perceived abandonment (in Maddie's case, discharge). Now that the discharge process is complete, suicidality will likely fade, and the usefulness of lithium becomes questionable, especially in light of its potential adverse effects.

B. Discontinue quetiapine. She was sleeping fine prior to hospitalization, so it is unlikely she will need it for long in the outpatient setting. [2] One would expect that quetiapine can be safely discontinued in the near future. The lack of preexisting insomnia and Maddie's interest in returning to school bode well for her baseline sleep pattern to assert itself now that she is out of the hospital.

C. Discontinue quetiapine. Patients should not be prescribed antipsychotics to treat insomnia. [2] It is also true that quetiapine is not a first-line agent to treat insomnia—whether or not the patient has BPD (Wilson et al. 2010).

D. No change, with a goal to continue this regimen. [3] Continuing medication need not be the goal—there is no research clearly indicating that medication (of any kind) should be continued in patients with BPD, whether indefinitely or for a specified duration.

E. No change, with a goal to discontinue one or both medications eventually. [1] Immediately following hospital discharge, providers will want to use whatever interventions are already in place to maximize the patient's emotional stability. Hence, the first appointment after discharge is probably not the best time to change medication for an adolescent with BPD.

Principles and clinical pearls for decision point 5:

- When patients try medications a second time, they and their providers may learn that whatever harm or benefit was attributed to the medication initially was misattributed and does not repeat itself. Misattribution is an easy trap to fall into when moods and behavior fluctuate often, but changes in BPD symptoms are as often coincidental with medication changes as they are a result of them.
- Medications that are effective in hospital settings often do not seem to provide the same benefit after discharge because both patients' environments and their mental states differ greatly in inpatient compared with outpatient care.
- Although the GPM model does allow that antipsychotic medication may be useful temporarily in a crisis, insomnia is not the symptom one should target (Gunderson and Links 2014). Moreover, Maddie has no baseline insomnia, indicating that sedating medication may be unnecessary once the disruptive situation changes. Hence, your goal should be to discontinue quetiapine, ideally over a period of 2–4 weeks.

6. What issue(s) regarding Maddie's hospitalization do you want to be sure to address?

A. Encourage a targeted family discussion about specific actions Maddie's parents can take to support her when she feels overwhelmed or suicidal. [1] We rely on parents to reduce adolescents' access to lethal means of suicide, including prescription and nonprescription medications. Parents can also be involved in developing or improving a safety plan. Further, they often can help adolescents access or practice coping skills.

B. Make a verbal or written agreement that she will contact you first if in the future she again feels the desire to overdose. [3] *Contracting for safety*, as these types of agreements are often called, is ineffective. It can undermine trust and offers no legal protection should a patient complete suicide or be injured when attempting.

The act of making and following through on a contract requires rational thought, which is not available to adolescents in the throes of suicidal urges. Hence, an adolescent who fails to adhere to a safety contract may feel like a failure, as if they have disappointed the provider. Importantly, research examining safety contracts has found that they do not prevent suicide or suicide attempts (Rudd et al. 2006). On the basis of such research, medical-legal experts recommend that providers *not* make contracts for safety, whether written or verbal.

C. Look back with Maddie at the events leading up to her overdose to find opportunities where she could have coped in other ways. [1] GPM-A advises providers to work with patients on clarifying precipitants whenever there is a genuine suicide attempt. GPM-A assumes that interpersonal stress or a loss of support will have occurred at some point in the day or days leading up to an attempt. Patients may not immediately recall such events or may inadvertently minimize their impact, so providers should ask patients explicitly and in detail about interpersonal stressors.

D. Be sure Maddie acknowledges that hospitalization only encourages regression; she should make better use of her crisis plan. [2] It may be broadly true that hospitalization reduces agency by taking care of people in situations where we wish they could take care of themselves. Certainly, we also can always encourage patients to put more effort into their own care. Nonetheless, GPM-A encourages providers to have a practical focus. Working collaboratively with patients, look closely at why they did not use a crisis plan effectively and what specific changes would ensure effective coping in the future.

E. Reflect with Maddie and her parents about whether her hospitalization indicates that the current treatment is not effective and should stop. [1] In GPM-A, providers should step back to reassess the effectiveness of treatment at specific time points, but another important opportunity for feedback is any time there is clinical deterioration, such as with hospitalization. The patient, the parents, and the provider may each have valuable insight into what is working in the current approach and what is not. When treatment is not working and a more effective approach cannot be found, that treatment should be stopped—regardless of the availability of other potential treatments.

Principles and clinical pearls for decision point 6:

- In the interpersonal hypersensitivity model, suicidal thoughts and actions result as a rapid reaction to interpersonal loss or withdrawal. The reactivity of this process means that understanding the events leading up to a hospitalization often reveals several opportunities to rapidly reverse that crash should a similar situation arise in the future. Hence, a chain analysis or similar review process may prevent subsequent hospitalizations.

- Contracting for safety in whatever form is not a clinically or legally appropriate intervention. Adolescents engage in self-harm and attempt suicide out of desperation; they are not capable of keeping a promise not to do so while they are feeling desperate. Similarly, it is counterproductive to ask for adolescents' word that they will contact you before attempting suicide. Especially when following the approach of GPM-A, in which we encourage patients to *not* rely on the clinician for their safety, it will benefit patients' agency if patients are encouraged to plan and use skills for effective coping.

- Parents may sometimes overreact to the prospect of their child attempting suicide, becoming terrified and hypervigilant, or they may underreact, having lived through so many episodes of self-harm and suicidal threats that they dismiss all of it as "attention-seeking" (clinicians may be guilty of that sometimes, too). Neither terror nor dismissiveness, however, are particularly compatible with effective, caring collaboration with the adolescent. Clinicians have an important opportunity to educate parents, both about the most likely drivers of suicidal behavior and about what practical steps they can take in the face of strong fear. Clinicians should encourage parents to connect empathically when adolescents express suicidality and also to prompt independent coping efforts and to set simple expectations for how they will respond to talk about suicide. For example: "If you say you want to kill yourself, I will take that seriously. I will bring you to the hospital or call 911."

7. How would you manage Maddie's medication regimen in light of this new complication?

   A. Prescribe appetite-suppressing medication such as luraglutide to counteract appetite increase from quetiapine. [3] There is no compelling argument to facilitate quetiapine use by adding an appetite-lowering medication because there is little justification to begin with to prescribe antipsychotic medication to adolescents with BPD.

B. No change: some people gain weight while taking antipsychotics, but 7% of body weight is not much and she may not gain any more. [2] Weight gain while taking antipsychotic medication is generally recognized as clinically significant when it exceeds 5%–7% of baseline body weight (e.g., McEvoy et al. 2007).

C. Discontinue quetiapine and check in after 2 weeks to see how she is doing. [1] GPM encourages providers to use medication briefly then discontinue it when the situation is more stable. Moreover, this degree of weight gain could by itself be a valid reason to discontinue quetiapine. A lower threshold could be considered for patients who are already overweight or obese.

D. Offer her and her parents psychoeducation about weight gain (e.g., managing caloric intake, portion control, purchasing healthy foods, limiting snacks). [2] Quetiapine might be continued if several conditions are met: 1) the patient strongly desires to continue, 2) weight gain does not exceed 7% of baseline weight, 3) the patient tolerates existing weight gain, 4) the patient and parents understand and implement psychoeducation about antipsychotic-related weight gain, and 5) the patient is willing to undergo recommended blood testing to monitor for any adverse metabolic effects.

E. Discontinue quetiapine and replace it with clonidine to be sure insomnia does not return. [2] Adding clonidine may be unnecessary. GPM principles encourage monitoring after providers discontinue medication. Providers can then prescribe new medication if the situation demands it, but not prophylactically.

Principles and clinical pearls for decision point 7:

- International guidelines recommend periodic blood tests to monitor metabolic function in patients taking antipsychotics (Pringsheim et al. 2011; www.camesaguideline.org). This recommendation is sometimes ignored, but it should be followed regardless of the patient's diagnosis. Patients who have a significant blood or needle phobia may decline to take antipsychotics; in GPM, especially for adolescents, such refusal is welcome because it eases the task of avoiding medication use as much as possible. For patients with such phobia who are willing to get their blood drawn, it is reasonable to offer a small, single dose of an anxiolytic—even a short-acting benzodiazepine—on an as-needed basis for the day of the blood draw. If patients do not get a blood test because they decline the anxiolytic or do not respond well, document this information to explain the absence of recommended testing.

- It is well in keeping with the case management model of GPM to bring up nutrition as a topic for discussion when treating an adolescent with BPD if it relates to a patient goal or directly to treatment. Thus, nutrition may be especially important to discuss with patients with disordered eating, those taking antipsychotic medication, and those whose weight is unhealthy (too high or too low).
- Weight gain due to antipsychotic medication is all too common. This adverse effect can be emphasized to patients and families when such medication is initially considered. Emphasis on the likelihood of weight gain can help meet two goals: First, it can set appropriate expectations for patients who do take such medication. Second, for patients and families worried about weight gain, knowing this risk can shift a conversation about solving problems with pills to one about solving problems with skills.

8. Would you make any changes to Maddie's medication regimen at this point?

   A. No change: she has not had stable function long enough to justify that. [2] There is no evidence to suggest that patients with BPD should remain on medication indefinitely. This is even more true for adolescents. Without research to guide clinical practice, providers treating adolescents with BPD may decide on a case-by-case basis how long of a period of stability is sufficient to begin work on discontinuing medication(s).

   B. Taper and discontinue lamotrigine. You expect this will destabilize Maddie emotionally, but you hope it will help her trust that you are listening to her needs. [1] A discontinuation trial will presumably strengthen a patient's trust in the provider. Strengthening trust is often a good reason in and of itself to recommend a medication change for some patients. The GPM model assumes medication will not reduce symptoms markedly; therefore, one would not expect the discontinuation of lamotrigine to lead the patient to decompensate.

   C. No change: although Maddie is functioning well, she can continue to take lamotrigine safely for a long time. [3] Even if the long-term safety of lamotrigine could be predicted, the GPM model aims to avoid long-term use.

   D. Taper and discontinue lamotrigine; no evidence supports long-term medication use, plus Maddie has demonstrated a meaningful period of emotional resilience. [1] Clinicians practicing GPM should attempt to discontinue medication for adolescents with stable function. Adolescents' chronological and developmental age and skills will factor in to choosing when that is appropriate. In this case, Maddie demonstrated 9 months of stable academic, social, and family functioning; at her age, that is long enough to try discontinuing lamotrigine.

E. Switch to an SSRI because SSRIs are safe for long-term use and you can avoid even a remote risk of Maddie developing Stevens-Johnson syndrome. [3] Switching to an SSRI might provide no benefit whatsoever. Furthermore, in the GPM model, you should consider using a new medication only after lamotrigine has been discontinued. You might choose an SSRI, but only if the symptoms somehow favor the properties of SSRIs over other medication classes.

Principles and clinical pearls for decision point 8:

- In GPM, medication use is viewed as temporary: it is meant to address pressing issues of the moment and then to be discontinued once the need is gone. Among patients with BPD who seem to benefit from ongoing medication use, a trial of a reduced dose or of discontinuation should still at least be attempted on a periodic basis. Importantly, this underscores to patients that they can expect that their skills and relationships will be sufficient to help them manage their symptoms.

- Because the evidence base for prescribing medication to adolescents with BPD is even weaker than that for adults, there may be times when, in the service of building rapport, it is therapeutic to acquiesce to a patient's or parent's strongly held desire about taking or not taking a particular medication at a particular dose. Such collaboration must of course be limited to what the prescribing provider deems is safe and appropriate overall—for example, allowing input from patients and/or families regarding the management of antidepressants or antipsychotics.

- Trauma is common among patients with BPD. When patients are ready, it is therapeutic to address the sequelae of trauma within the framework of GPM. Although trauma can have a major impact on attachment relationships, the focus in adolescent GPM on "school before love" targets academic performance before the impacts of trauma. As this case demonstrates, providers can do that effectively, providing case management–based treatment without first tackling trauma or trauma-related symptoms. When trauma is eventually addressed in GPM, the integrative philosophy of GPM allows providers to use therapeutic techniques of all kinds, including mentalizing, cognitive-behavioral skills, and exposure.

References

Abraham PF, Calabrese JR: Evidenced-based pharmacologic treatment of border-line personality disorder: a shift from SSRIs to anticonvulsants and atypical antipsychotics? J Affect Disord 111(1):21–30, 2008 18304647

Adler KA, Finch EF, Rodriguez-Villa AM, Choi-Kain LW: Primary care providers, in Applications of Good Psychiatric Management for Borderline Personality Disorder: A Practical Guide. Edited by Choi-Kain LW, Gunderson JG. Washington, DC, American Psychiatric Association Publishing, 2019, pp 169–186

Agrawal HR, Gunderson J, Holmes BM, et al: Attachment studies with borderline patients: a review. Harv Rev Psychiatry 12(2):94–104, 2004 15204804

Al-Mateen CS, Jones K, Linker J, et al: Clinician response to a child who completes suicide. Child Adolesc Psychiatr Clin N Am 27(4):621–635, 2018 30219223

American Academy of Child and Adolescent Psychiatry (AACAP) Committee on Telepsychiatry and AACAP Committee on Quality Issues: Clinical update: telepsychiatry with children and adolescents. J Am Acad Child Adolesc Psychiatry 56(10):875–893, 2017 28942810

American Psychiatric Association: Practice Guideline for the Treatment of Patients With Borderline Personality Disorder. Washington, DC, American Psychiatric Publishing, 2001

American Psychiatric Association: Diagnostic and Statistical Manual of Mental Disorders, 5th Edition. Arlington, VA, American Psychiatric Publishing, 2013

Amminger GP, Chanen AM, Ohmann S, et al: Omega-3 fatty acid supplementation in adolescents with borderline personality disorder and ultra-high risk criteria for psychosis: a post hoc subgroup analysis of a double-blind, randomized controlled trial. Can J Psychiatry 58(7):402–408, 2013 23870722

Andrewes HE, Hulbert C, Cotton SM, et al: An ecological momentary assessment investigation of complex and conflicting emotions in youth with borderline personality disorder. Psychiatry Res 252:102–110, 2017 28259033

Andrewes HE, Hulbert C, Cotton SM, et al: Patterns of non-suicidal self-injury and their relationship with suicide attempts in youth with borderline personality disorder. Arch Suicide Res 22(3):465–478, 2018 28759336

Andrewes HE, Hulbert C, Cotton SM, et al: Relationships between the frequency and severity of non-suicidal self-injury and suicide attempts in youth with borderline personality disorder. Early Interv Psychiatry 13(2):194–201, 2019 28718985

Antonovsky A: The salutogenic model as a theory to guide health promotion. Health Promot Int 11(1):11–18, 1996

Asaad T, Okasha T, Okasha A: Sleep EEG findings in ICD-10 borderline personality disorder in Egypt. J Affect Disord 71(1–3):11–18, 2002 12167496

Bagge C, Nickell A, Stepp S, et al: Borderline personality disorder features predict negative outcomes 2 years later. J Abnorm Psychol 113(2):279–288, 2004 15122948

Bagge CL, Stepp SD, Trull TJ: Borderline personality disorder features and utilization of treatment over two years. J Pers Disord 19(4):420–439, 2005 16178683

Bailey RC, Grenyer BF: Supporting a person with personality disorder: a study of carer burden and well-being. J Pers Disord 28(6):796–809, 2014 16178683

Bailey RC, Grenyer BF: The relationship between expressed emotion and wellbeing for families and carers of a relative with borderline personality disorder. Personal Ment Health 9(1):21–32, 2015 25195577

Bandelow B, Krause J, Wedekind D, et al: Early traumatic life events, parental attitudes, family history, and birth risk factors in patients with borderline personality disorder and healthy controls. Psychiatry Res 134(2):169–179, 2005 15840418

Bateman A: Treating borderline personality disorder in clinical practice. Am J Psychiatry 169(6):560–563, 2012 22684591

Bateman A, Fonagy P: Effectiveness of partial hospitalization in the treatment of borderline personality disorder: a randomized controlled trial. Am J Psychiatry 156(10):1563–1569, 1999 10518167

Bateman A, Fonagy P: Mentalization-Based Treatment for Personality Disorders: A Practical Guide. Oxford, UK, Oxford University Press, 2016

Bayes AJ, Parker GB: Differentiating borderline personality disorder (BPD) from bipolar disorder: diagnostic efficiency of DSM BPD criteria. Acta Psychiatr Scand 141(2):142–148, 2020 31758547

Beck E, Bo S, Gondan M, et al: Mentalization-based treatment in groups for adolescents with borderline personality disorder (BPD) or subthreshold BPD versus treatment as usual (M-GAB): study protocol for a randomized controlled trial. Trials 17(1):1–3, 2016 27405522

Bender DS, Skodol AE, Pagano ME, et al: Prospective assessment of treatment use by patients with personality disorders. Psychiatr Serv 57(2):254–257, 2006 16452705

Benton SA, Robertson JM, Tseng WC, et al: Changes in counseling center client problems across 13 years. Prof Psychol Res Pract 34(1):66–72, 2003

Bernstein DP, Cohen P, Velez CN, et al: Prevalence and stability of the DSM-III-R personality disorders in a community-based survey of adolescents. Am J Psychiatry 150(8):1237–1243, 1993 8328570

Biskin RS: Treatment of borderline personality disorder in youth. J Can Acad Child Adolesc Psychiatry 22(3):230–234, 2013 23970912

Black DW, Blum N, Pfohl B, et al: Suicidal behavior in borderline personality disorder: prevalence, risk factors, prediction, and prevention. J Pers Disord 18(3):226–239, 2004 15237043

Bleiberg E: The clinical challenge of children and adolescents with severe personality disorders. Bull Menninger Clin 54(1):107–120, 1989 2302468

Blum N, St John D, Pfohl B, et al: Systems Training for Emotional Predictability and Problem Solving (STEPPS) for outpatients with borderline personality disorder: a randomized controlled trial and 1-year follow-up. Am J Psychiatry 165(4):468–478, 2008 18281407

Bo S, Sharp C, Beck E, et al: First empirical evaluation of outcomes for mentalization-based group therapy for adolescents with BPD. Personal Disord 8(4):396–401, 2017 27845526

Bo S, Vilmar JW, Jensen SL, et al: What works for adolescents with borderline personality disorder: towards a developmentally informed understanding and structured treatment model. Curr Opin Psychol 37:7–12, 2020 32652486

Bohus M, Dyer AS, Priebe K, et al: Dialectical behaviour therapy for post-traumatic stress disorder after childhood sexual abuse in patients with and without borderline personality disorder: a randomised controlled trial. Psychother Psychosom 82(4):221–233, 2013 23712109

Bohus M, Kleindienst N, Hahn C, et al: Dialectical behavior therapy for posttraumatic stress disorder (DBT-PTSD) compared with cognitive processing therapy (CPT) in complex presentations of PTSD in women survivors of childhood sexual abuse. JAMA Psychiatry July 22, 2020 Epub ahead of print 32697288

Boritz T, Barnhart R, McMain SF: The influence of posttraumatic stress disorder on treatment outcomes of patients with borderline personality disorder. J Pers Disord 30(3):395–407, 2016 26305394

Bornovalova MA, Verhulst B, Webber T, et al: Genetic and environmental influences on the codevelopment among borderline personality disorder traits, major depression symptoms, and substance use disorder symptoms from adolescence to young adulthood. Dev Psychopathol 30(1):49–65, 2018 28420454

Bozzatello P, Rocca P, De Rosa ML, et al: Current and emerging medications for borderline personality disorder: is pharmacotherapy alone enough? Expert Opin Pharmacother 21(1):47–61, 2020 31693423

Brand S, Kirov R: Sleep and its importance in adolescence and in common adolescent somatic and psychiatric conditions. Int J Gen Med 4:425–442, 2011 21731894

Bridler R, Häberle A, Müller ST, et al: Psychopharmacological treatment of 2195 in-patients with borderline personality disorder: a comparison with other psychiatric disorders. Eur Neuropsychopharm 25(6):763–772, 2015 25907249

Brown RC, Plener PL: Non-suicidal self-injury in adolescence. Curr Psychiatry Rep 19(3):20, 2017 28315191

Buckholdt KE, Parra GR, Jobe-Shields L: Intergenerational transmission of emotion dysregulation through parental invalidation of emotions: implications for adolescent internalizing and externalizing behaviors. J Child Fam Stud 23(2):324–332, 2014 24855329

Buitron V, Hill RM, Pettit JW, et al: Interpersonal stress and suicidal ideation in adolescence: an indirect association through perceived burdensomeness toward others. J Affect Disord 190:143–149, 2016 26519633

Burnett S, Sebastian C, Cohen Kadosh K, et al: The social brain in adolescence: evidence from functional magnetic resonance imaging and behavioural studies. Neurosci Biobehav Rev 35(8):1654–1664, 2011 21036192

Cailhol L, Jeannot M, Rodgers R, et al: Borderline personality disorder and mental healthcare service use among adolescents. J Pers Disord 27(2):252–259, 2013 23514188

Cairns KE, Yap MB, Pilkington PD, et al: Risk and protective factors for depression that adolescents can modify: a systematic review and meta-analysis of longitudinal studies. J Affect Disord 169:61–75, 2014 25154536

Calvo N, Lara B, Serrat L, et al: The role of environmental influences in the complex relationship between borderline personality disorder and attention-deficit/hyperactivity disorder: review of recent findings. Borderline Personal Disord Emot Dysregul 7:2, 2020 31921426

Carter G, Page A, Large M, et al: Royal Australian and New Zealand College of Psychiatrists clinical practice guideline for the management of deliberate self-harm. Aust New Zeal J Psychiatry 50(10):939–1000, 2016 27650687

Cartwright M, Wardle J, Steggles N, et al: Stress and dietary practices in adolescents. Health Psychol 22(4):362–369, 2003 12940392

Chanen AM, Kaess M: Developmental pathways to borderline personality disorder. Curr Psychiatry Rep 14(1):45–53, 2012 22009682

Chanen AM, McCutcheon L: Prevention and early intervention for borderline personality disorder: current status and recent evidence. Br J Psychiatry 54:s24–s29 2013, 23288497

Chanen AM, Thompson K: Preventive strategies for borderline personality disorder in adolescents. Current Treatment Options in Psychiatry 1(4):358–368, 2014

Chanen AM, Thompson K: Borderline personality and mood disorders: risk factors, precursors, and early signs in childhood and youth, in Borderline Personality and Mood Disorders: Comorbidity and Controversy. Edited by Choi-Kain LW, Gunderson JG. New York, Springer, 2015, pp 155–174

Chanen AM, Thompson KN: The age of onset of personality disorders, in Age of Onset of Mental Disorders: Etiopathogenetic and Treatment Implications. Edited by de Girolamo G, McGorry PD, Sartorius N. Cham, Switzerland, Springer International, 2019, pp 183–201

Chanen AM, Jackson HJ, McGorry PD, et al: Two-year stability of personality disorder in older adolescent outpatients. J Pers Disord 18(6):526–541, 2004 15615665

Chanen AM, Jovev M, Jackson HJ: Adaptive functioning and psychiatric symptoms in adolescents with borderline personality disorder. J Clin Psychiatry 68(2):297–306, 2007 17335330

Chanen AM, Jackson HJ, McCutcheon LK, et al: Early intervention for adolescents with borderline personality disorder using cognitive analytic therapy: randomised controlled trial. Br J Psychiatry 193(6):477–484, 2008a 19043151

Chanen AM, Jovev M, Djaja D, et al: Screening for borderline personality disorder in outpatient youth. J Pers Disord 22:353–364, 2008b 18684049

Chanen A, Jovev M, McCutcheon L, et al: Borderline personality disorder in young people and the prospects for prevention and early intervention. Curr Psychiatry Rev 4(1):48–57, 2008c

Chanen AM, McCutcheon LK, Germano D, et al: The HYPE Clinic: an early intervention service for borderline personality disorder. J Psychiatr Pract 15(3):163–172, 2009 19461389

Chanen AM, McCutcheon L, Kerr IB: HYPE: a cognitive analytic therapy-based prevention and early intervention programme for borderline personality disorder, in Handbook of Borderline Personality Disorder in Children and Adolescents. Edited by Tackett JL, Sharp C. New York, Springer, 2014, pp 361–383

Chanen AM, Berk M, Thompson K: Integrating early intervention for borderline personality disorder and mood disorders. Harv Rev Psychiatry 24(5):330–341, 2016 27144298

Chanen A, Sharp C, Hoffman P, et al: Prevention and early intervention for borderline personality disorder: a novel public health priority. World Psychiatry 16(2):215–216, 2017 28498598

Chanen AM, Nicol K, Betts JK, et al: Diagnosis and treatment of borderline personality disorder in young people. Curr Psychiatry Rep 22(5):25, 2020 32335771

Choi-Kain LW, Gunderson JG (eds): Borderline Personality and Mood Disorders: Comorbidity and Controversy. New York, Springer, 2015

Choi-Kain LW, Gunderson JG (eds): Applications of Good Psychiatric Management for Borderline Personality Disorder. Washington, DC, American Psychiatric Association Publishing, 2019

Choi-Kain LW, Fitzmaurice GM, Zanarini MC, et al: The relationship between self-reported attachment styles, interpersonal dysfunction, and borderline personality disorder. J Nerv Ment Dis 197(11):816–821, 2009 19996719

Choi-Kain LW, Albert EB, Gunderson JG: Evidence-based treatments for borderline personality disorder: implementation, integration, and stepped care. Harv Rev Psychiatry 24(5):342–356, 2016 27603742

Choudhury S, Blakemore SJ, Charman T: Social cognitive development during adolescence. Soc Cogn Affect Neurosci 1(3):165–174, 2006 18985103

Chu BC, Rizvi SL, Zendegui EA, et al: Dialectical behavior therapy for school refusal: treatment development and incorporation of web-based coaching. Cogn Behav Pract 22(3):317–330, 2015

Cloud J: Borderline personality: the disorder doctors fear the most. Time, January 8, 2009. Available at: http://content.time.com/time/subscriber/article/0,33009,1870491-3,00.html. Accessed September 15, 2020.

Cohen P, Crawford TN, Johnson JG, et al: The children in the community study of developmental course of personality disorder. J Pers Disord 19(5):466–486, 2005 16274277

Cohen GL, Prinstein MJ: Peer contagion of aggression and health risk behavior among adolescent males: an experimental investigation of effects on public conduct and private attitudes. Child Dev 77(4):967–983, 2006 16942500

Conway CC, Hipwell AE, Stepp SD: Seven-year course of borderline personality disorder features: borderline pathology is as unstable as depression during adolescence. Clin Psychol Sci 5(4):742–749 2017 28920008

Cooney EB, Davis KL, Thompson P, et al: Feasibility of evaluating DBT for self-harming adolescents: a small randomised controlled trial. Auckland, Te Pou o Te Whakaaro Nui, New Zealand Mental Health Research, August 2010. Available at: www.tepou.co.nz/uploads/files/resource-assets/feasibility-of-evaluating-dbt-for-self-harming-adolescents.pdf. Accessed September 15, 2020.

Cooney E, Davis K, Thompson P, et al: Feasibility of comparing dialectical behavior therapy with treatment as usual for suicidal and self-injuring adolescents: follow-up data from a small randomized controlled trial, in Is DBT Effective With Multi-Problem Adolescents? Show Me the Data! An International Presentation of Three Randomized Trials Evaluating DBT With Adolescents. Miller AL (Chair). Symposium conducted at the Annual Meting of the Association of Behavioral and Cognitive Therapies, National Harbor, MD, November 15–18, 2012

Courtney DB, Makinen J: Impact of diagnosis disclosure on adolescents with borderline personality disorder. J Can Acad Child Adolesc Psychiatry 25(3):177–184, 2016 27924148

Crawford MJ, Sanatinia R, Barrett B, et al: Lamotrigine for people with borderline personality disorder: a RCT. Health Technol Assess 22(17):1–68, 2018 29651981

Crawford TN, Cohen P, Brook J: Dramatic-erratic personality disorder symptoms I: continuity from early adolescence into adulthood. J Pers Disord 15(4):319–335, 2001 11556699

Crick NR, Murray-Close D, Woods K: Borderline personality features in childhood: a short-term longitudinal study. Dev Psychopathol 17(4):1051–1070, 2005 16613430

Cristea IA, Gentili C, Cotet CD, et al: Efficacy of psychotherapies for borderline personality disorder: a systematic review and meta-analysis. JAMA Psychiatry 74(4):319–328, 2017 28249086

Daly AM, Llewelyn S, McDougall E, et al: Rupture resolution in cognitive analytic therapy for adolescents with borderline personality disorder. Psychol Psychother 83(Pt 3):273–288, 2010 20109279

Darling N: Participation in extracurricular activities and adolescent adjustment: cross-sectional and longitudinal findings. J Youth Adolesc 34(5):493–505, 2005 de Haan AM, Boon AE, de Jong JT, et al: Therapeutic relationship and dropout in youth mental health care with ethnic minority children and adolescents. Clinical Psychologist 18(1):1–9, 2014

Desrosiers L, Saint-Jean M, Breton JJ: Treatment planning: a key milestone to prevent treatment dropout in adolescents with borderline personality disorder. Psychol Psychother 88(2):178–196, 2015 24957784

Desrosiers L, Saint-Jean M, Laporte L, et al: Engagement complications of adolescents with borderline personality disorder: navigating through a zone of turbulence. Borderline Personal Disord Emot Dysregul 7:18, 2020 32884818

Distel MA, Trull TJ, Derom CA, et al: Heritability of borderline personality disorder features is similar across three countries. Psychol Med 38(9):1219–1229, 2008 17988414

Dixon-Gordon KL, Chapman AL, Lovasz N, et al: Too upset to think: the interplay of borderline personality features, negative emotions and social problem solving in the laboratory. Personal Disord 2(4):243–260, 2011 22448801

Driessens CM: Extracurricular activity participation moderates impact of family and school factors on adolescents' disruptive behavioural problems. BMC Public Health 15:1110, 2015 26558510

Egger HL, Costello EJ, Angold A: School refusal and psychiatric disorders: a community study. J Am Acad Child Adolesc Psychiatry 42:797–807, 2003 12819439

Eisler I, Dare C, Hodes M, et al: Family therapy for adolescent anorexia nervosa: the results of a controlled comparison of two family interventions. J Child Psychol Psychiatry 41(6):727–736, 2000 11039685

Erikson EH: Growth and crises of the "healthy personality," in Symposium on the Healthy Personality. Edited by Senn MJE. New York, Josiah Macy, Jr, Foundation, 1950, pp 91–146

Ferrer M, Andión O, Matalí J, et al: Comorbid attention-deficit/hyperactivity disorder in borderline patients defines an impulsive subtype of borderline personality disorder. J Pers Disord 24(6):812–822, 2010 21158602

Firth J, Torous J, Nicholas J, et al: The efficacy of smartphone-based mental health interventions for depressive symptoms: a meta-analysis of randomized controlled trials. World Psychiatry 16(3):287–298, 2017 28941113

Flynn D, Kells M, Joyce M, et al: Family connections versus optimised treatment-as-usual for family members of individuals with borderline personality disorder: non-randomised controlled study. Borderline Personal Disord Emot Dysregul 4:18, 2017 28861273

Fonagy P, Allison E: The role of mentalizing and epistemic trust in the therapeutic relationship. Psychotherapy (Chic) 51(3):372–380, 2014 24773092

Fonagy P, Campbell C: Mentalizing, attachment and epistemic trust: how psychotherapy can promote resilience. Psychiatr Hung 32(3):283–287, 2017 29135441

Fonagy P, Speranza M, Luyten P, et al: ESCAP Expert Article: borderline personality disorder in adolescence: an expert research review with implications for clinical practice. Eur Child Adolesc Psychiatry 24(11):1307–1320, 2015 26271454

Fonagy P, Luyten P, Allison E, et al: What we have changed our minds about: part 1. Borderline personality disorder as a limitation of resilience. Borderline Personal Disord Emot Dysregul 4:11, 2017 28413687

Fonagy P, Luyten P, Allison E, et al: Mentalizing, epistemic trust and the phenomenology of psychotherapy. Psychopathology 52(2):94–103, 2019 31362289

Fossati A: Diagnosing borderline personality disorder in adolescence: a review of the published literature. Scand J Child Adolesc Psychiatr Psychol 3(1):5–21, 2015

Fossati A, Gratz KL, Maffei C, et al: Impulsivity dimensions, emotion dysregulation, and borderline personality disorder features among Italian nonclinical adolescents. Borderline Personal Disord Emot Dysregulation 1:5, 2014 26401289

Fox KR, Franklin JC, Ribeiro JD, et al: Meta-analysis of risk factors for nonsuicidal self-injury. Clin Psychol Rev 42:156–167, 2015 26416295

Franklin JC, Hessel ET, Aaron RV, et al: The functions of nonsuicidal self-injury: support for cognitive-affective regulation and opponent processes from a novel psychophysiological paradigm. J Abnorm Psychol 119(4):850–862, 2010 20939652

Fristad MA, Arnett MM, Gavazzi SM: The impact of psychoeducational workshops on families of mood-disordered children. Family Therapy 25(3):151–159, 1998

Fruzzetti AE, Shenk C, Hoffman PD: Family interaction and the development of borderline personality disorder: a transactional model. Dev Psychopathol 17(4):1007–1030, 2005 16613428

Gabbard GO: Do all roads lead to Rome? New findings on borderline personality disorder. Am J Psychiatry 164(6):853–855, 2007 17541040

Garland AF, Lewczyk-Boxmeyer CM, Gabayan EN, et al: Multiple stakeholder agreement on desired outcomes for adolescents' mental health services. Psychiatr Serv 55(6):671–676, 2004 15175465

Geller B, Luby J: Child and adolescent bipolar disorder: a review of the past 10 years. J Am Acad Child Adolesc Psychiatry 36(9):1168–1176, 1997 9291717

Gersh E, Hulbert CA, McKechnie B, et al: Alliance rupture and repair processes and therapeutic change in youth with borderline personality disorder. Psychol Psychother 90(1):84–104, 2017 27240265

Ghinea D, Koenig J, Parzer P, et al: Longitudinal development of risk-taking and self-injurious behavior in association with late adolescent borderline personality disorder symptoms. Psychiatry Res 273:127–133, 2019 30641342

Giffin J: Family experience of borderline personality disorder. Aust N Z J Fam Ther 29(3):133–138, 2008

Giletta M, Burk WJ, Scholte RH, et al: Direct and indirect peer socialization of adolescent nonsuicidal self-injury. J Res Adolesc 23(3):450–463, 2013 26412955

Glenn CR, Klonsky ED: Prospective prediction of nonsuicidal self-injury: a 1-year longitudinal study in young adults. Behav Ther 42(4):751–762, 2011 22036002

Glenn CR, Klonsky ED: Nonsuicidal self-injury disorder: an empirical investigation in adolescent psychiatric patients. J Clin Child Adolesc Psychol 42:496–507, 2013 23682597

Gobbi G, Atkin T, Zytynski T, et al: Association of cannabis use in adolescence and risk of depression, anxiety, and suicidality in young adulthood: a systematic review and meta-analysis. JAMA Psychiatr 76(4):426–434, 2019 30758486

Goldfried MR: Obtaining consensus in psychotherapy: what holds us back? Am Psychol 74(4):484–496, 2019 30221947

Golubchik P, Sever J, Zalsman G, et al: Methylphenidate in the treatment of female adolescents with cooccurrence of attention deficit/hyperactivity disorder and borderline personality disorder: a preliminary open-label trial. Int Clin Psychopharmacol 23(4):228–231, 2008 18446088

Goodman M, Patil U, Triebwasser J, et al: Parental burden associated with borderline personality disorder in female offspring. J Pers Disord 25(1):59–74, 2011 21309623

Goodman M, Perez-Rodriguez MM, Siever L: The neurobiology of adolescent-onset borderline personality disorder, in Handbook of Borderline Personality Disorder in Children and Adolescents. Edited by Tackett JL, Sharp C. New York, Springer, 2014, pp 113–128

Goodman M, Tomas IA, Temes CM, et al: Suicide attempts and self-injurious behaviours in adolescent and adult patients with borderline personality disorder. Personal Ment Health 11:157–163, 2017 28544496

Gottfried MA: Chronic absenteeism and its effects on students' academic and socioemotional outcomes. Journal of Education Students Placed at Risk 19(2):53–75, 2014

Granic I, Dishion TJ: Deviant talk in adolescent friendships: a step toward measuring a pathogenic attractor process. Soc Dev 12(3):314–334, 2003

Grant BF, Chou SP, Goldstein RB, et al: Prevalence, correlates, disability, and comorbidity of DSM-IV borderline personality disorder: results from the Wave 2 National Epidemiologic Survey on Alcohol and Related Conditions. J Clin Psychiatry 69(4):533–545, 2008 18426259

Gratz KL, Berghoff CR, Richmond JR, et al: Examining posttraumatic stress disorder as a predictor of treatment response to dialectical behavior therapy. J Clin Psychol 76(9):1563–1574, 2020 32445601

Greenfield B, Henry M, Lis E, et al: Correlates, stability and predictors of borderline personality disorder among previously suicidal youth. Eur Child Adolesc Psychiatry 24(4):397–406, 2015 25084977

Griffiths M: Validity, utility and acceptability of borderline personality disorder diagnosis in childhood and adolescence: survey of psychiatrists. Psychiatrist 35(1):19–22, 2011

Grilo CM, Sanislow CA, Gunderson JG, et al: Two-year stability and change of schizotypal, borderline, avoidant, and obsessive-compulsive personality disorders. J Consult Clin Psychol 72(5):767–775, 2004 15482035

Grilo CM, Stout RL, Markowitz JC, et al: Personality disorders predict relapse after remission from an episode of major depressive disorder: a 6-year prospective study. J Clin Psychiatry 71(12):1629–1635, 2010 20584514

Groschwitz RC, Plener PL, Kaess M, et al: The situation of former adolescent self-injurers as young adults: a follow-up study. BMC Psychiatry 15:160, 2015 26187150

Gunderson JG: Borderline Personality Disorder. Washington, DC, American Psychiatric Press, 1984

Gunderson JG: The borderline patient's intolerance of aloneness: insecure attachments and therapist availability. Am J Psychiatry 153(6):752–758, 1996 8633685

Gunderson JG: Disturbed relationships as a phenotype for borderline personality disorder. Am J Psychiatry 164(11):1637–1640, 2007 17974925

Gunderson JG: Borderline Personality Disorder: A Clinical Guide, 2nd Edition. Washington, DC, American Psychiatric Publishing, 2008

Gunderson JG, Berkowitz C: A BPD brief: an introduction to borderline personality disorder. New York, National Education Alliance for Borderline Personality Disorder, 2006a. Available at: www.borderlinepersonalitydisorder.org/professionals/a-bpd-brief. Accessed September 15, 2020.

Gunderson JG, Berkowitz C: Family guidelines: multiple family group program at McLean Hospital. Belmont, MA, New England Personality Disorder Association, 2006b. Available at: www.borderlinepersonalitydisorder.org/family connections/family guidelines. Accessed September 15, 2020.

Gunderson JG, Choi-Kain LW: Medication management for patients with borderline personality disorder. Am J Psychiatry 175(8):709–711, 2018 30064243

Gunderson JG, Links P: Borderline Personality Disorder: A Clinical Guide, 2nd Edition. Washington, DC, American Psychiatric Publishing, 2008

Gunderson JG, Links P: Handbook of Good Psychiatric Management for Borderline Personality Disorder. Washington, DC, American Psychiatric Publishing, 2014

Gunderson JG, Lyons-Ruth K: BPD's interpersonal hypersensitivity phenotype: a gene-environment-developmental model. J Pers Disord 22(1):22–41, 2008 18312121

Gunderson JG, Palmer BA: Inpatient psychiatric units, in Applications of Good Psychiatric Management for Borderline Personality Disorder: A Practical Guide. Edited by Choi-Kain LW, Gunderson JG. Washington, DC, American Psychiatric Association Publishing, 2019, pp 11–36

Gunderson JG, Shea MT, Skodol AE, et al: The Collaborative Longitudinal Personality Disorders Study: development, aims, design, and sample characteristics. J Pers Disord 14(4):300–315, 2000 11213788

Gunderson JG, Bender D, Sanislow C, et al: Plausibility and possible determinants of sudden "remissions" in borderline patients. Psychiatry 66(2):111–119, 2003 12868289

Gunderson JG, Morey LC, Stout RL, et al: Major depressive disorder and borderline personality disorder revisited: longitudinal interactions. J Clin Psychiatry 65(8):1049–1056, 2004 15323588

Gunderson JG, Daversa MT, Grilo CM, et al: Predictors of 2-year outcome for patients with borderline personality disorder. Am J Psychiatry 163(5):822–826, 2006 16648322

Gunderson JG, Stout RL, McGlashan TH, et al: Ten-year course of borderline personality disorder: psychopathology and function from the Collaborative Longitudinal Personality Disorders Study. Arch Gen Psychiatry 68(8):827–837, 2011a 21464343

Gunderson JG, Zanarini MC, Choi-Kain LW, et al: Family study of borderline personality disorder and its sectors of psychopathology. Arch Gen Psychiatry 68(7):753–762, 2011b 21727257

Gunderson JG, Stout RL, Shea MT, et al: Interactions of borderline personality disorder and mood disorders over 10 years. J Clin Psychiatry 75(8):829–834, 2014 25007118

Gunderson JG, Herpertz SC, Skodol AE, et al: Borderline personality disorder. Nat Rev Dis Primers 4:18029, 2018 29795363

Gutheil TG: Suicide, suicide litigation, and borderline personality disorder. J Pers Disord 18:248–256, 2004 15237045

Ha C, Balderas JC, Zanarini MC, et al: Psychiatric comorbidity in hospitalized adolescents with borderline personality disorder. J Clin Psychiatry 75(5):e457–e464, 2014 24922498

Hahlweg K, Goldstein MJ, Nuechterlein KH, et al: Expressed emotion and patient-relative interaction in families of recent-onset schizophrenics. J Consult Clin Psychol 57(1):11–18, 1989 2925960

Hamza CA, Stewart SL, Willoughby T: Examining the link between nonsuicidal self-injury and suicidal behavior: a review of the literature and an integrated model. Clin Psychol Rev 32:482–495, 2012 22717336

Harned MS, Chapman AL, Dexter-Mazza ET, et al: Treating co-occurring axis I disorders in recurrently suicidal women with borderline personality disorder: a 2-year randomized trial of dialectical behavior therapy versus community treatment by experts. J Consult Clin Psychol 76(6):1068–1075, 2008 19045974

Harned MS, Jackson SC, Comtois KA, et al: Dialectical behavior therapy as a precursor to PTSD treatment for suicidal and/or self-injuring women with borderline personality disorder. J Trauma Stress 23(4):421–429, 2010 20648564

Harned MS, Korslund KE, Linehan MM: A pilot randomized controlled trial of dialectical behavior therapy with and without the dialectical behavior therapy prolonged exposure protocol for suicidal and self-injuring women with borderline personality disorder and PTSD. Behav Res Ther 55:7–17, 2014 24562087

Harned MS, Wilks CR, Schmidt SC, et al: Improving functional outcomes in women with borderline personality disorder and PTSD by changing PTSD severity and post-traumatic cognitions. Behav Res Ther 103:53–61, 2018 29448136

Hasking P, Whitlock J, Voon D, et al: A cognitive-emotional model of NSSI: using emotion regulation and cognitive processes to explain why people self-injure. Cogn Emot 31(8):1543–1556, 2017 27702245

Hawton K, Witt KG, Salisbury TL, et al: Interventions for self-harm in children and adolescents. Cochrane Database Syst Rev (12):CD012013, 2015 26688129

Hazen E, Schlozman S, Beresin E: Adolescent psychological development: a review. Pediatr Rev 29(5):161–167, 2008 18450837

Hennings JM: Function and psychotherapy of chronic suicidality in borderline personality disorder: using the reinforcement model of suicidality. Front Psychiatry 11:99, 2020 32256412

Hermens ML, van Splunteren PT, van den Bosch A, et al: Barriers to implementing the clinical guideline on borderline personality disorder in the Netherlands. Psychiatr Serv 62(11):1381–1383, 2011 22211222

Heron M: Deaths: leading causes for 2017. Natl Vital Stat Rep 68(6):1–77, 2019 32501203

Herpertz SC, Bertsch K: The social-cognitive basis of personality disorders. Curr Opin Psychiatry 27(1):73–77, 2014 24270477

Hersh RG: Assessment and treatment of patients with borderline personality disorder in the college and university population. J College Stud Psychother 27(4):304–322, 2013

Hersh RG: Integration with transference-focused psychotherapy, in Applications of Good Psychiatric Management for Borderline Personality Disorder. Edited by Choi-Kain LW, Gunderson JG. Washington, DC, American Psychiatric Association Publishing, 2019, pp 37–56

Hill RM, Penner F, Vanwoerden S, et al: Interpersonal trust and suicide ideation among adolescent psychiatric inpatients: an indirect effect via perceived burdensomeness. Suicide Life Threat Behav 49(1):240–252, 2019 29370447

Ho J, Panagiotopoulos C, McCrindle B, et al: Management recommendations for metabolic complications associated with second-generation antipsychotic use in children and youth. J Can Acad Child Adolesc Psychiatry 20(3):234–241, 2011 21804854

Hoffman PD, Fruzzetti A, Swenson C: Dialectical behavior therapy-family skills training. Fam Process 38(4):399–414, 1999 10668619

Hoffman PD, Fruzzetti AE, Buteau E, et al: Family connections: a program for relatives of persons with borderline personality disorder. Fam Process 44(2):217–225, 2005 16013747

Hong V: Borderline personality disorder in the emergency department: good psychiatric management. Harv Rev Psychiatry 24(5):357–366, 2016 27603743

Hong V: Emergency departments, in Applications of Good Psychiatric Management for Borderline Personality Disorder. Edited by Choi-Kain LW, Gunderson JG. Washington, DC, American Psychiatric Association Publishing, 2019, pp 37–56

Honig A, Hofman A, Rozendaal N, et al: Psycho-education in bipolar disorder: effect on expressed emotion. Psychiatry Res 72(1):17–22, 1997 7568553

Hooley JM: Expressed emotion and depression, in Depression and Families: Impact and Treatment. Edited by Keitner GI. Washington, DC, American Psychiatric Press, 1990, pp 57–83

Hooley JM: Expressed emotion and relapse of psychopathology. Annu Rev Clin Psychol 3:329–352, 2007 17716059

Hooley JM, Franklin JC: Why do people hurt themselves? A new conceptual model of nonsuicidal self-injury. Clin Psychol Sci 6(3):428–451, 2018

Hutsebaut J, Videler AC, Verheul R, et al: Managing borderline personality disorder from a life course perspective: clinical staging and health management. Personal Disord 10(4):309–316, 2019 31144839

Huỳnh C, Guilé J-M, Breton J-J, et al: Sleep-wake patterns of adolescents with borderline personality disorder and bipolar disorder. Child Psychiatry Hum Dev 47(2):202–214, 2016 26003420

Iliakis EA, Sonley AK, Ilagan GS, et al: Treatment of borderline personality disorder: is supply adequate to meet public health needs? Psychiatr Serv 70(9):772–781, 2019 31138059

Ingenhoven TJ, Duivenvoorden HJ: Differential effectiveness of antipsychotics in borderline personality disorder: meta-analyses of placebo-controlled, randomized clinical trials on symptomatic outcome domains. J Clin Psychopharmacol 31(4):489–496, 2011 21694626

James AC, Vereker M: Family therapy for adolescents diagnosed as having borderline personality disorder. J Fam Ther 18(3):269–283, 1996

Johnson JG, Cohen P, Skodol AE, et al: Personality disorders in adolescence and risk of major mental disorders and suicidality during adulthood. Arch Gen Psychiatry 56(9):805–811, 1999 12884886

Johnson JG, Cohen P, Kasen S, et al: Age-related change in personality disorder trait levels between early adolescence and adulthood: a community-based longitudinal investigation. Act Psychiatr Scand 102(4):265–275, 2000 11089726

Johnson JG, Cohen P, Kasen S, et al: Cumulative prevalence of personality disorders between adolescence and adulthood. Acta Psychiatr Scand 118(5):410–413, 2008 18644003

Johnston LD, Miech RA, O'Malley PM, et al: Monitoring the Future National Survey Results on Drug Use, 1975–2017: Overview, Key Findings on Adolescent Drug Use. Ann Arbor, MI, Institute for Social Research, University of Michigan, 2018

Jopling EN, Khalid-Khan S, Chandrakumar SF, et al: A retrospective chart review: adolescents with borderline personality disorder, borderline personality traits, and controls. Int J Adolesc Med Health 30(2), 2016 27442360

Jørgensen MS, Storebø OJ, Simonsen E: Systematic review and meta-analyses of psychotherapies for adolescents with subclinical and borderline personality disorder: methodological issues. Can J Psychiatry 65(1):59–60, 2020 31813274

Jovev M, Green M, Chanen A, et al: Attentional processes and responding to affective faces in youth with borderline personality features. Psychiatry Res 199(1):44–50, 2012 22503381

Kaess M, Brunner R, Chanen A: Borderline personality disorder in adolescence. Pediatrics 134(4):782–793, 2014 25246626

Kaess M, Fischer-Waldschmidt G, Resch F, et al: Health related quality of life and psychopathological distress in risk taking and self-harming adolescents with full-syndrome, subthreshold and without borderline personality disorder: rethinking the clinical cut-off? Borderline Personal Disord Emot Dysregul 4:7, 2017 28484600

Kalpakci A, Venta A, Sharp C: Beliefs about unmet interpersonal needs mediate the relation between conflictual family relations and borderline personality features in young adult females. Borderline Personal Disord Emot Dysregulation 1:11, 2014 26401295

Kasen S, Cohen P, Chen H, et al: School climate and continuity of adolescent personality disorder symptoms. J Child Psychol Psychiatry 50:1504–1512, 2009 19573031

Kazdin AE: Dropping out of child psychotherapy: issues for research and implications for practice. Clin Child Psychol Psychiatry 1(1):133–156, 1996

Kendler KS, Prescott CA, Myers J, et al: The structure of genetic and environmental risk factors for common psychiatric and substance use disorders in men and women. Arch Gen Psychiatry 60(9):929–937, 2003 12963675

Kendler KS, Myers J, Reichborn-Kjennerud T: Borderline personality disorder traits and their relationship with dimensions of normative personality: a web-based cohort and twin study. Acta Psychiatr Scand 123(5):349–359, 2011 21198457

Kernberg OF: Suicidal behavior in borderline patients: diagnosis and psychotherapeutic considerations. Am J Psychother 47(2):245–254, 1993 8517472

Kessler RC, Avenevoli S, McLaughlin KA, et al: Lifetime co-morbidity of DSM-IV disorders in the US National Comorbidity Survey Replication Adolescent Supplement (NCS-A). Psychol Med 42(9):1997–2010, 2012 22273480

Keuroghlian AS, Gunderson JG, Pagano ME, et al: Interactions of borderline personality disorder and anxiety disorders over 10 years. J Clin Psychiatry 76(11):1529–1534, 2015 26114336

Keuroghlian AS, Palmer BA, Choi-Kain LW, et al: The effect of attending good psychiatric management (GPM) workshops on attitudes towards patients with borderline personality disorder. J Pers Disord 30(4):567–576, 2016 26111249

Kim EY, Miklowitz DJ: Expressed emotion as a predictor of outcome among bipolar patients undergoing family therapy. J Affect Disord 82(3):343–352, 2004 15555685

Kitzrow MA: The mental health needs of today's college students: challenges and recommendations. NASPA Journal 41(1):167–181, 2003

Kolla NJ, Eisenberg H, Links PS: Epidemiology, risk factors, and psychopharmacological management of suicidal behavior in borderline personality disorder. Arch Suicide Res 12(1):1–19, 2008 18240030

Kolla NJ, Links PS, McMain S, et al: Demonstrating adherence to guidelines for the treatment of patients with borderline personality disorder. Can J Psychiatry 54(3):181–189, 2009 19321022

Kolly S, Despland JN, de Roten Y, et al: Therapist adherence to good psychiatric practice in a short-term treatment for borderline personality disorder. J Nerv Ment Dis 204(7):489–493, 2016 27787770

Kothgassner OD, Robinson K, Goreis A, et al: Does treatment method matter? A meta-analysis of the past 20 years of research on therapeutic interventions for self-harm and suicidal ideation in adolescents. Borderline Personality Disord Emot Dysregul 7:1–6, 2020 32426138

Kramer U, Berger T, Kolly S, et al: Effects of motive-oriented therapeutic relationship in early phase treatment of borderline personality disorder: a pilot study of a randomized trial. J Nerv Ment Dis 199(4):244–250, 2011 21451348

Kramer U, Kolly S, Berthoud L, et al: Effects of motive-oriented therapeutic relationship in a ten-session general psychiatric treatment of borderline personality disorder: a randomized controlled trial. Psychother Psychosom 83(3):176–186, 2014

Kramer U, Stulz N, Berthoud L, et al: The shorter the better? A follow-up analysis of 10-session psychiatric treatment including the motive-oriented therapeutic relationship for borderline personality disorder. Psychother Res 27(3):362–370, 2017a 26684670

Kramer U, Temes CM, Magni LR, et al: Psychosocial functioning in adolescents with and without borderline personality disorder. Personal Ment Health 11(3):164–170, 2017b 28597585

Krischer M, Ponton-Rodriguez T, Gooran GR, et al: Transference focused psychotherapy for borderline-adolescents in a day clinic treatment program [in German]. Praxis Kinderpsychol Kinderpsychiatr 66(6):445–464, 2017 28701090

Kuja-Halkola R, Juto KL, Skoglund C, et al: Do borderline personality disorder and attention-deficit/hyperactivity disorder co-aggregate in families? A population-based study of 2 million Swedes. Mol Psychiatry 15:1–9, 2018 30233291

Laporte L, Paris J, Guttman H, et al: Psychopathology, childhood trauma, and personality traits in patients with borderline personality disorder and their sisters. J Pers Disord 25(4):448–462, 2011 21838561

Laurenssen EM, Hutsebaut J, Feenstra DJ, et al: Diagnosis of personality disorders in adolescents: a study among psychologists. Child Adolesc Psychiatry Ment Health 7(1):3, 2013 23398887

Laurenssen EM, Hutsebaut J, Feenstra DJ, et al: Feasibility of mentalization-based treatment for adolescents with borderline symptoms: a pilot study. Psychotherapy (Chic) 51(1):159–166, 2014 24059741

Lawn S, McMahon J: Experiences of family carers of people diagnosed with borderline personality disorder. J Psychiatr Ment Health Nurs 22(4):234–243, 2015 25857849

Lazarus SA, Beardslee J, Pedersen SL, et al: A within-person analysis of the association between borderline personality disorder and alcohol use in adolescents. J Abnorm Child Psychol 45(6):1157–1167, 2017 27812907

Lazarus SA, Choukas-Bradley S, Beeney JE, et al: Too much too soon? Borderline personality disorder symptoms and romantic relationships in adolescent girls. J Abnorm Child Psychol 47(12):1995–2005, 2019 31240430

Lee NK, Cameron J, Jenner L: A systematic review of interventions for co-occurring substance use and borderline personality disorders. Drug Alcohol Rev 34(6):663–672, 2015 25919396

Lester R, Prescott L, McCormack M, et al: Service users' experiences of receiving a diagnosis of borderline personality disorder: a systematic review. Personal Ment Health 14(3)263–283, 2020 32073223

Leung SW, Leung F: Construct validity and prevalence rate of borderline personality disorder among Chinese adolescents. J Pers Disord 23(5):494–513, 2009 19817630

Levy KN, Becker DF, Grilo CM, et al: Concurrent and predictive validity of the personality disorder diagnosis in adolescent inpatients. Am J Psychiatry 156(10):1522–1528, 1999 10518161

Linehan MM, Armstrong HE, Suarez A, et al: Cognitive-behavioral treatment of chronically parasuicidal borderline patients. Arch Gen Psychiatry 48:1060–1064, 1991 18455222

Links PS, Gould B, Ratnayake R: Assessing suicidal youth with antisocial, borderline, or narcissistic personality disorder. Can J Psychiatry 48(5):301–310, 2003 12866335

Lloyd-Richardson EE, Perrine N, Dierker L, et al: Characteristics and functions of non-suicidal self-injury in a community sample of adolescents. Psychol Med 37(8):1183–1192, 2007 17349105

Loas G, Pham-Scottez A, Cailhol L, et al: Axis II comorbidity of borderline personality disorder in adolescents. Psychopathology 46(3):172–175, 2013 23006475

Lubans D, Richards J, Hillman C, et al: Physical activity for cognitive and mental health in youth: a systematic review of mechanisms. Pediatrics 138(3):e20161642, 2016 27542849

Luyten P, Campbell C, Allison E, et al: The mentalizing approach to psychopathology: state of the art and future directions. Annu Rev Clin Psychol 16:297–325, 2020 32023093

Maltsberger JT, Ronningstam E, Weinberg I, et al: Suicide fantasy as a life-sustaining recourse. J Am Acad Psychoanal Dyn Psychiatry 38(4):611–623, 2010 21171902

Marchant A, Hawton K, Stewart A, et al: A systematic review of the relationship between internet use, self-harm and suicidal behaviour in young people: the good, the bad and the unknown. PLoS One 12(8):e0181722, 2017 28813437

Mars B, Heron J, Klonsky ED, et al: Predictors of future suicide attempt among adolescents with suicidal thoughts or non-suicidal self-harm: a population-based birth cohort study. Lancet Psychiatry 6(4):327–337, 2019 30879972

Marttunen MJ, Aro HM, Henriksson MM, et al: Mental disorders in adolescent suicide. DSM-III-R axes I and II diagnoses in suicides among 13- to 19-year-olds in Finland. Arch Gen Psychiatry 48(9):834–839, 1991 1929774

Masland SR, Price D, MacDonald J, et al: Enduring effects of one-day training in good psychiatric management on clinician attitudes about borderline personality disorder. J Nerv Ment Dis 206(11):865–869, 2018 30371640

Masland SR, Cummings MH, Null KE, et al: Changes in post-traumatic stress disorder symptoms during residential treatment for borderline personality disorder: a longitudinal cross-lagged study. Borderline Personal Disord Emot Dysregul 6:15, 2019 31719988

Mason MJ, Schmidt C, Abraham A, et al: Adolescents' social environment and depression: social networks, extracurricular activity, and family relationship influences. J Clin Psychol Med Settings 16(4):346–354, 2009 19621251

McCauley E, Berk MS, Asarnow JR, et al: Efficacy of dialectical behavior therapy for adolescents at high risk for suicide: a randomized clinical trial. JAMA Psychiatry 75(8):777–785, 2018 29926087

McEvoy JP, Lieberman JA, Perkins DO, et al: Efficacy and tolerability of olanzapine, quetiapine, and risperidone in the treatment of early psychosis: a randomized, double-blind 52-week comparison. Am J Psychiatry 164(7):1050–1060, 2007 17606657

McGlashan TH, Grilo CM, Skodol AE, et al: The Collaborative Longitudinal Personality Disorders Study: baseline axis I/II and II/II diagnostic co-occurrence. Acta Psychiatr Scand 102(4):256–264, 2000 11089725

McMain SF, Links PS, Gnam WH, et al: A randomized trial of dialectical behavior therapy versus general psychiatric management for borderline personality disorder. Am J Psychiatry 166(12):1365–1374, 2009 19755574

McMain SF, Guimond T, Streiner DL, et al: Dialectical behavior therapy compared with general psychiatric management for borderline personality disorder: clinical outcomes and functioning over a 2-year follow-up. Am J Psychiatry 169(6):650–661, 2012 22581157

Mehlum L, Tørmoen AJ, Ramberg M, et al: Dialectical behavior therapy for adolescents with repeated suicidal and self-harming behavior: a randomized trial. J Am Acad Child Adolesc Psychiatry 53(10):1082–1091, 2014 25245352

Mehlum L, Ramberg M, Tørmoen AJ, et al: Dialectical behavior therapy compared with enhanced usual care for adolescents with repeated suicidal and self-harming behavior: outcomes over a one-year follow-up. J Am Acad Child Adolesc Psychiatry 55(4):295–300, 2016 27015720

Mehlum L, Ramleth RK, Tørmoen AJ, et al: Long term effectiveness of dialectical behavior therapy versus enhanced usual care for adolescents with self-harming and suicidal behavior. J Child Psychol Psychiatry 60(10):1112–1122, 2019 31127612

Mercer D, Douglass AB, Links PS: Meta-analyses of mood stabilizers, antidepressants and antipsychotics in the treatment of borderline personality disorder: effectiveness for depression and anger symptoms. J Pers Disord 23(2):156–174, 2009 19379093

Mercer D, Links PS, Sonley AKI, et al: Integration with dialectical behavior therapy, in Applications of Good Psychiatric Management for Borderline Personality Disorder. Edited by Choi-Kain LW, Gunderson JG. Washington, DC, American Psychiatric Association Publishing, 2019, pp 37–56

Midgley N, Holmes J, Parkinson S, et al: "Just like talking to someone about like shit in your life and stuff, and they help you": hopes and expectations for therapy among depressed adolescents. Psychother Res 26(1):11–21, 2016 25372575

Miller CJ, Flory JD, Miller SR, et al: Childhood attention-deficit/hyperactivity disorder and the emergence of personality disorders in adolescence: a prospective follow-up study. J Clin Psychiatry 69(9):1477–1484, 2008 19193347

Morales-Muñoz I, Broome MR, Marwaha S: Association of parent-reported sleep problems in early childhood with psychotic and borderline personality disorder symptoms in adolescence. JAMA Psychiatry July 1, 2020 Epub ahead of print 32609357

Moran P, Coffey C, Romaniuk H, et al: The natural history of self-harm from adolescence to young adulthood: a population-based cohort study. Lancet 379(9812):236–243, 2012 22100201

Morey LC: Personality Assessment Inventory (PAI): Professional Manual. Lutz, FL, Psychological Assessment Resources, 2007

Myers K, Nelson EL, Rabinowitz T, et al: American Telemedicine Association practice guidelines for telemental health with children and adolescents. Telemed J E Health 23(10):779–804, 2017 28930496

Nadort M, Arntz A, Smit JH, et al: Implementation of outpatient schema therapy for borderline personality disorder with versus without crisis support by the therapist outside office hours: a randomized trial. Behav Res Ther 47(11):961–973, 2009 19698939

Noblin JL, Venta A, Sharp C: The validity of the MSI-BPD among inpatient adolescents. Assessment 21(2):210–217, 2014 23344914

Nock MK: Self-injury. Annu Rev Clin Psychol 6:339–363, 2010 20192787

Nock MK, Prinstein MJ: Contextual features and behavioral functions of self-mutilation among adolescents. J Abnorm Psychol 114(1):140–146, 2005 15709820

Nock MK, Joiner TE Jr, Gordon KH, et al: Non-suicidal self-injury among adolescents: diagnostic correlates and relation to suicide attempts. Psychiatry Res 144(1):65–72, 2006 16887199

Nock MK, Prinstein MJ, Sterba SK: Revealing the form and function of self-injurious thoughts and behaviors: a real-time ecological assessment study among adolescents and young adults. J Abnorm Psychol 118(4):816–827, 2009 19899851

Nook EC, Sasse SF, Lambert HK, et al: The nonlinear development of emotion differentiation: granular emotional experience is low in adolescence. Psychol Sci 29(8):1346–1357, 2018 29878880

Normandin L, Ensink K, Kernberg OF: Transference-focused psychotherapy for borderline adolescents: a neurobiologically informed psychodynamic psychotherapy. J Infant Child Adolesc Psychother 14(1):98–110, 2015

Nosè M, Cipriani A, Biancosino B, et al: Efficacy of pharmacotherapy against core traits of borderline personality disorder: meta-analysis of randomized controlled trials. Int Clin Psychopharmacol 21(6):345–353, 2006 17012981

Oberle E, Ji XR, Guhn M, et al: Benefits of extracurricular participation in early adolescence: associations with peer belonging and mental health. J Youth Adolesc 48(11):2255–2270, 2019 31440881

O'Keeffe S, Martin P, Target M, et al: "I just stopped going": a mixed methods investigation into types of therapy dropout in adolescents with depression. Front Psychol 10:75, 2019 30804827

Orme W, Bowersox L, Vanwoerden S, et al: The relation between epistemic trust and borderline pathology in an adolescent inpatient sample. Borderline Personal Disord Emot Dysregulation 6:13, 2019 31485332

Ougrin D, Tranah T, Stahl D, et al: Therapeutic interventions for suicide attempts and self-harm in adolescents: systematic review and meta-analysis. J Am Acad Child Adolesc Psychiatry 54(2):97.e2–107.e2, 2015 25617250

Packman WL, O'Connor Pennuto T, Bongar B, et al: Legal issues of professional negligence in suicide cases. Behav Sci Law 22(5):697–713, 2004 15378596

Paris J: Is hospitalization useful for suicidal patients with borderline personality disorder? J Pers Disord 18(3):240–247, 2004 15237044

Paris J: Stepped care: an alternative to routine extended treatment for patients with borderline personality disorder. Psychiatr Serv 64(10):1035–1037, 2013 23945913

Paris J: A history of research on borderline personality disorder in childhood and adolescence, in Handbook of Borderline Personality Disorder in Children and Adolescents. Edited by Sharp C, Tackett JL. New York, Springer, 2014, pp 9–16

Paris J, Zweig-Frank H: A 27-year follow-up of patients with borderline personality disorder. Compr Psychiatry 42(6):482–487, 2001 11704940

Paris J, Perlin J, Laporte L, et al: Exploring resilience and borderline personality disorder: a qualitative study of pairs of sisters. Pers Ment Health 8(3):199–208, 2014 24700757

Pearce J, Jovev M, Hulbert C: Evaluation of a psychoeducational group intervention for family and friends of youth with borderline personality disorder. Borderline Personal Disord Emot Dysregul 4:5, 2017 28352470

Pennay A, Cameron J, Reichert T, et al: A systematic review of interventions for co-occurring substance use disorder and borderline personality disorder. J Subst Abuse Treat 41(4):363–373, 2011 21742460

Penner F, Wall K, Jardin C, et al: A study of risky sexual behavior, beliefs about sexual behavior, and sexual self-efficacy in adolescent inpatients with and without borderline personality disorder. Personal Disord Theory 10(6):524–535, 2019 31259605

Plante DT, Zanarini MC, Frankenburg FR, et al: Sedative-hypnotic use in patients with borderline personality disorder and axis II comparison subjects. J Pers Disord 23(6):563–571, 2009 20001175

Plener PL, Schumacher TS, Munz LM, et al: The longitudinal course of non-suicidal self-injury and deliberate self-harm: a systematic review of the literature. Borderline Personal Disord Emot Dysregul 2:2, 2015 26401305

Plener PL, Brunner R, Fegert JM, et al: Treating nonsuicidal self-injury (NSSI) in adolescents: consensus based German guidelines. Child Adolesc Psychiatry Ment Health 10:46, 2016 27933099

Pompili M, Girardi P, Ruberto A, et al: Suicide in borderline personality disorder: a meta-analysis. Nord J Psychiatry 59(5):319–324, 2005 16757458

Poreh AM, Rawlings D, Claridge G, et al: The BPQ: a scale for the assessment of borderline personality based on DSM-IV criteria. J Pers Disord 20(3):247–260, 2006 16776554

Price D: Generalist adult outpatient psychiatry practice, in Applications of Good Psychiatric Management for Borderline Personality Disorder. Edited by Choi-Kain LW, Gunderson JG. Washington, DC, American Psychiatric Association Publishing, 2019, pp 85–116

Pringsheim T, Panagiotopoulos C, Davidson J, Ho J; Canadian Alliance for Monitoring Effectiveness and Safety of Antipsychotics in Children (CAMESA) guideline group: Evidence-based recommendations for monitoring safety of second generation antipsychotics in children and youth. Paediatr Child Health 16(9):581–589, 2011 23115502

Prinstein MJ, Heilbron N, Guerry JD, et al: Peer influence and nonsuicidal self-injury: longitudinal results in community and clinically referred adolescent samples. J Abnorm Child Psychol 38(5):669–862, 2010 20437255

Project Air: You've been diagnosed with BPD—what now? Wollongong, NSW, Australia, Project Air Strategy for Personality Disorders, University of Wollongong, 2020. Available at: www.projectairstrategy.org/content/groups/public/@web/@project-air/documents/doc/uow260274.pdf. Accessed September 12, 2020.

Rasmussen KG: Do patients with personality disorders respond differentially to electroconvulsive therapy? A review of the literature and consideration of conceptual issues. J ECT 31(1):6–12, 2015 25054362

Rathus JH, Miller AL: Dialectical behavior therapy adapted for suicidal adolescents. Suicide Life Threat Behav 32(2):146–157, 2002 12079031

Rathus JH, Miller AL: DBT Skills Manual for Adolescents. New York, Guilford, 2014

Reich DB, Zanarini MC, Bieri KA: A preliminary study of lamotrigine in the treatment of affective instability in borderline personality disorder. Int Clin Psychopharmacol 24:270–275, 2009 19636254

Reitz S, Kluetsch R, Niedtfeld I, et al: Incision and stress regulation in borderline personality disorder: neurobiological mechanisms of self-injurious behaviour. Br J Psychiatry 207(2):165–172, 2015 25906795

Reuter TR, Sharp C, Temple JR, et al: The relation between borderline personality disorder features and teen dating violence. Psychol Violence 5(2):163–173, 2015

Rich CL, Runeson BS: Similarities in diagnostic comorbidity between suicide among young people in Sweden and the United States. Acta Psychiatr Scand 86(5):335–339, 1992 1485522

Rickard N, Arjmand HA, Bakker D, et al: Development of a mobile phone app to support self-monitoring of emotional well-being: a mental health digital innovation. JMIR Ment Health 3(4):e49, 2016 27881358

Ridolfi ME, Rossi R, Occhialini G, et al: A clinical trial of a psychoeducation group intervention for patients with borderline personality disorder. J Clin Psychiatry 81(1):19m12753, 2019 31917907

Robinson K, Garisch JA, Kingi T, et al: Reciprocal risk: the longitudinal relationship between emotion regulation and non-suicidal self-injury in adolescents. J Abnorm Child Psychol 47(2):325–332, 2019 29923162

Rodman AM, Powers KE, Somerville LH: Development of self-protective biases in response to social evaluative feedback. Proc Natl Acad Sci USA 114(50):13,158–13,163, 2017 29180428

Rossouw TI, Fonagy P: Mentalization-based treatment for self-harm in adolescents: a randomized controlled trial. J Am Acad Child Adolesc Psychiatry 51(12):1304–1313, 2012 23200287

Rudd MD, Mandrusiak M, Joiner TE Jr: The case against no-suicide contracts: the commitment to treatment statement as a practice alternative. J Clin Psychol 62(2):243–251, 2006 16342293

Runeson B, Beskow J: Borderline personality disorder in young Swedish suicides. J Nerv Ment Dis 179(3):153–156, 1991 1997663

Sadeh N, Londahl-Shaller EA, Piatigorsky A, et al: Functions of non-suicidal self-injury in adolescents and young adults with borderline personality disorder symptoms. Psychiatry Res 216(2):217–222, 2014 24594204

Sakinofsky I: The aftermath of suicide: managing survivors' bereavement. Can J Psychiatry 52(6 suppl 1):129S–136S, 2007 17824358

Sansone RA, Levitt JL, Sansone LA: The prevalence of personality disorders among those with eating disorders. Eat Disord 13(1):7–21, 2004 16864328

Scalzo F, Hulbert CA, Betts JK: Substance use in youth with borderline personality disorder. J Pers Disord 32(5):603–617, 2018 28926304

Schaefer DR, Simpkins SD, Vest AE, et al: The contribution of extracurricular activities to adolescent friendships: new insights through social network analysis. Dev Psychol 47(4):1141–1152, 2011 21639618

Schmahl C, Bohus M, Esposito F, et al: Neural correlates of antinociception in borderline personality disorder. Arch Gen Psychiatry 63(6):659–666, 2006 16754839

Schulze L, Schmahl C, Niedtfeld I: Neural correlates of disturbed emotion processing in borderline personality disorder: a multimodal meta-analysis. Biol Psychiatry 79(2):97–106, 2016 25935068

Schuppert HM, Giesen-Bloo J, van Gemert TG, et al: Effectiveness of an emotion regulation group training for adolescents—a randomized controlled pilot study. Clin Psychol Psychother 16(6):467–478, 2009 19630069

Schuppert HM, Timmerman ME, Bloo J, et al: Emotion regulation training for adolescents with borderline personality disorder traits: a randomized controlled trial. J Am Acad Child Adolesc Psychiatry 51(12):1314–1323, 2012 23200288

Scott LN, Pilkonis PA, Hipwell AE, et al: Non-suicidal self-injury and suicidal ideation as predictors of suicide attempts in adolescent girls: a multi-wave prospective study. Compr Psychiatry 58:1–10, 2015 25595520

Sekowski M, Gambin M, Sharp C: The relations between identity disturbances, borderline features, internalizing disorders, and suicidality in inpatient adolescents. J Pers Disord Jan 21, 2021 33779274 Epub ahead of print

Shanks C, Pfohl B, Blum N, et al: Can negative attitudes toward patients with borderline personality disorder be changed? The effect of attending a STEPPS workshop. J Pers Disord 25(6):806–812, 2011 22217226

Sharp C: The social-cognitive basis of BPD: a theory of hypermentalizing, in Handbook of Borderline Personality Disorder in Children and Adolescents. Edited by Tackett JL, Sharp C. New York, Springer, 2014, pp 211–225

Sharp C: Calling for a unified redefinition of "borderlineness": commentary on Gunderson et al. J Pers Disord 32(2):168–174, 2018 29561721

Sharp C: Editorial: What's in a name? The importance of adolescent personality pathology for adaptive psychosocial function. J Am Acad Child Adolesc Psychiatry 59(10):1130–1132, 2020 31654694

Sharp C, Fonagy P: Practitioner review: borderline personality disorder in adolescence—recent conceptualization, intervention, and implications for clinical practice. J Child Psychol Psychiatry 56(12):1266–1288, 2015 26251037

Sharp C, Wall K: Personality pathology grows up: adolescence as a sensitive period. Curr Opin Psychol 21:111–116, 2018 29227834

Sharp C, Pane H, Ha C, et al: Theory of mind and emotion regulation difficulties in adolescents with borderline traits. J Am Acad Child Adolesc Psychiatry 50(6):563.e1–573.e1, 2011 21621140

Sharp C, Green KL, Yaroslavsky I, et al: The incremental validity of borderline personality disorder relative to major depressive disorder for suicidal ideation and deliberate self-harm in adolescents. J Pers Disord 26(6):927–938, 2012 23281677

Sharp C, Ha C, Carbone C, et al: Hypermentalizing in adolescent inpatients: treatment effects and association with borderline traits. J Pers Disord 27(1):3–18, 2013 23342954

Sharp C, Steinberg L, Temple J, et al: An 11-item measure to assess borderline traits in adolescents: refinement of the BPFSC using IRT. Personal Disord 5(1):70–78 2014 24588063

Sharp C, Wright AG, Fowler JC, et al: The structure of personality pathology: both general ('g') and specific ('s') factors? J Abnorm Psychol 124(2):387–398, 2015 25730515

Sharp C, Vanwoerden S, Wall K: Adolescence as a sensitive period for the development of personality disorder. Psychiatr Clin North Am 41(4):669–683, 2018 30447731

Sharp C, Vanwoerden S, Gallagher M, et al: The course of borderline psychopathology in adolescents with complex mental health problems: an 18 month longitudinal follow-up study. Res Child Adolesc Psychopathol 13:1–3 2021 33439418 Epub ahead of print

Shaw J: Adolescence, mourning and creativity. Adolesc Psychiatry 9:60–77, 1981 7340550

Shea MT, Stout RL, Yen S, et al: Associations in the course of personality disorders and axis I disorders over time. J Abnorm Pyschol 113(4):499–508, 2004 15535783

Shepherd A, Sanders C, Shaw J: Seeking to understand lived experiences of personal recovery in personality disorder in community and forensic settings—a qualitative methods investigation. BMC Psychiatry 17(1):282, 2017 28764672

Silk KR, Feurino L III: Psychopharmacology of personality disorders, in The Oxford Handbook of Personality Disorders. Edited by Widiger T. London, Oxford University Press, 2012, pp 712–726

Simoneau TL, Miklowitz DJ, Saleem R: Expressed emotion and interactional patterns in the families of bipolar patients. J Abnorm Psychol 107(3):497–507, 1998 9715584

Simonsen S, Bateman A, Bohus M, et al: European guidelines for personality disorders: past, present and future. Borderline Personal Disord Emot Dysregul 6:9, 2019 31143448

Skodol AE, Gunderson JG, McGlashan TH, et al: Functional impairment in patients with schizotypal, borderline, avoidant, or obsessive-compulsive personality disorder. Am J Psychiatry 159(2):276–283, 2002 11823271

Skodol AE, Johnson JG, Cohen P, et al: Personality disorder and impaired functioning from adolescence to adulthood. Br J Psychiatry 190(5):415–420, 2007 17470956

Soeteman DI, Hakkaart-van Roijen L, Verheul R, et al: The economic burden of personality disorders in mental health care. J Clin Psychiatry 69(2):259–265, 2008 18363454

Soloff PH, Chiappetta L: 10-year outcome of suicidal behavior in borderline personality disorder. J Pers Disord 33(1):82–100, 2019 29469667

Spielmans GI, Spence-Sing T, Parry P: Duty to warn: antidepressant black box suicidality warning is empirically justified. Front Psychiatry 11:18, 2020 32116839

Spirito A, Esposito-Smythers C, Wolff J, et al: Cognitive-behavioral therapy for adolescent depression and suicidality. Child Adolesc Psychiatr Clin N Am 20(2):191–204, 2011 21440850

Stepp SD, Trull TJ, Sher KJ: Borderline personality features predict alcohol use problems. J Pers Disord 19(6):711–722, 2005 16553564

Stepp SD, Keenan K, Hipwell AE, et al: The impact of childhood temperament on the development of borderline personality disorder symptoms over the course of adolescence. Borderline Personal Disord Emot Dysregul 1(1):18, 2014a 26064524

Stepp SD, Whalen DJ, Scott LN, et al: Reciprocal effects of parenting and borderline personality disorder symptoms in adolescent girls. Dev Psychopathol 26(2):361–378, 2014b 24443951

Stigler KA, Potenza MN, Posey DJ, et al: Weight gain associated with atypical antipsychotic use in children and adolescents: prevalence, clinical relevance, and management. Paediatr Drugs 6(1):33–44, 2004 14969568

Sulzer SH, Muenchow E, Potvin A, et al: Improving patient-centered communication of the borderline personality disorder diagnosis. J Ment Health 25(1):5–9, 2016 26360788

Swahn MH, West B, Bossarte RM: Urban girls and boys who date: a closer look at the link between dating and risk for alcohol and drug use, self-harm and suicide attempts. Vulnerable Children and Youth Studies 4(3):249–254, 2009

Swannell SV, Martin GE, Page A, et al: Prevalence of nonsuicidal self-injury in nonclinical samples: systematic review, meta-analysis and meta-regression. Suicide Life-Threatening Behav 44(3):273–303, 2014 24422986

Tackett JL, Balsis S, Oltmanns TF, et al: A unifying perspective on personality pathology across the life span: Developmental considerations for the fifth edition of the Diagnostic and Statistical Manual of Mental Disorders. Dev Psychopathol 21(3):687–713, 2009 19583880

Temes CM, Frankenburg FR, Fitzmaurice GM, et al: Deaths by suicide and other causes among patients with borderline personality disorder and personality-disordered comparison subjects over 24 years of prospective follow-up. J Clin Psychiatry 80(1):18m12436, 2019 30688417

Thompson KN, Betts J, Jovev M, et al: Sexuality and sexual health among female youth with borderline personality disorder pathology. Early Interv Psychiatry 13(3):502–508, 2019a 29076247

Thompson KN, Jackson H, Cavelti M, et al: The clinical significance of subthreshold borderline personality disorder features in outpatient youth. J Pers Disord 33(1):71–81, 2019b 30036169

Torgersen S, Myers J, Reichborn-Kjennerud T, et al: The heritability of cluster B personality disorders assessed both by personal interview and questionnaire. J Pers Disord 26(6):848–866, 2012 23281671

Tougas A-M, Rassy J, Frenette-Bergeron É, et al: "Lost in transition": a systematic mixed studies review of problems and needs associated with school reintegration after psychiatric hospitalization. School Ment Health 11:629–649, 2019

Tritt K, Nickel C, Lahmann C, et al: Lamotrigine treatment of aggression in female borderline patients: a randomized, double-blind, placebo-controlled study. J Psychopharmacol 19(3):287–291, 2005 15888514

Trull TJ, Useda JD, Conforti K, et al: Borderline personality disorder features in non-clinical young adults: 2. Two-year outcome. J Abnorm Psychol 106(2):307–314, 1997 9131850

Unruh BT, Sonley AKI, Choi-Kain LW: Integration with mentalization-based treatment, in Applications of Good Psychiatric Management for Borderline Personality Disorder. Edited by Choi-Kain LW, Gunderson JG. Washington, DC, American Psychiatric Association Publishing, 2019, pp 37–56

U.S. Food and Drug Administration: Suicidality in children and adolescents treated with antidepressant medications. Silver Spring, MD, U.S. Food and Drug Administration, February 5, 2018. Available at: www.fda.gov/drugs/postmarket-drug-safety-information-patients-and-providers/suicidality-children-and-adolescents-being-treated-antidepressant-medications. Accessed September 11, 2020.

Vanwoerden S, Leavitt J, Gallagher MW, et al: Dating violence victimization and borderline personality pathology: temporal associations from late adolescence to early adulthood. Personal Disord 10(2):132–142, 2019 30829527

Venta A, Magyar M, Hossein S, et al: The psychometric properties of the Personality Assessment Inventory–Adolescent's Borderline Features Scale across two high-risk samples. Psychol Assess 30(6):827, 2018 29469580

Vijay NR, Links PS: New frontiers in the role of hospitalization for patients with personality disorders. Curr Psychiatry Rep 9:63–67, 2007 17257516

Vita A, De Peri L, Sacchetti E: Antipsychotics, antidepressants, anticonvulsants, and placebo on the symptom dimensions of borderline personality disorder: a meta-analysis of randomized controlled and open-label trials. J Clin Psychopharmacol 31(5):613–624, 2011 21869691

von Ceumern-Lindenstjerna IA, Brunner R, Parzer P, et al: Attentional bias in later stages of emotional information processing in female adolescents with borderline personality disorder. Psychopathology 43(1):25–32, 2010 19893341

Wall K, Vanwoerden S, Penner F, et al: Adolescent sleep disturbance, emotion regulation and borderline features in an inpatient setting. J Clin Child Adolesc Psychol 43(1):1–15, 2020 32603239

Washburn JJ, Richardt SL, Styer DM, et al: Psychotherapeutic approaches to nonsuicidal self-injury in adolescents. Child Adolesc Psychiatry Ment Health 6(1):14, 2012 22463499

Weibel S, Nicastro R, Prada P, et al: Screening for attention-deficit/hyperactivity disorder in borderline personality disorder. J Affect Disord 226:85–91, 2018 28964997

Weinberg I, Maltsberger JT: Suicidal behavior in borderline personality disorder, in Suicide in Psychiatric Disorders. Edited by Tatarelli R, Pompili M, Girardi P. New York, Nova Science, 2007, pp 333–370

Weiner AS, Ensink K, Normandin L: Psychotherapy for borderline personality disorder in adolescents. Psychiatric Clinics 41(4):729–746, 2018 30447735

Wilcox HC, Arria AM, Caldeira KM, et al: Longitudinal predictors of past-year non-suicidal self-injury and motives among college students. Psychol Med 42(4):717–726, 2012 21906421

Williams TF, Scalco MD, Simms LJ: The construct validity of general and specific dimensions of personality pathology. Psychol Med 48(5):834–848, 2018 28826417

Wilson SJ, Nutt DJ, Alford C, et al: British Association for Psychopharmacology consensus statement on evidence-based treatment of insomnia, parasomnias and circadian rhythm disorders. J Psychopharmacol 24(11):1577–1601, 2010 20813762

Winnicott DW: Transitional objects and transitional phenomena—a study of the first not-me possession. Int J Psychoanal 34(2):89–97, 1953 13061115

Winograd G, Cohen P, Chen H: Adolescent borderline symptoms in the community: prognosis for functioning over 20 years. J Child Psychol Psychiatry 49(9):933–941, 2008 18665882

Winsper C, Tang NKY: Linkages between insomnia and suicidality: prospective associations, high-risk subgroups and possible psychological mechanisms. Int Rev Psychiatry 26(2):189–204, 2014 24892894

Winsper C, Marwaha S, Lereya ST, et al: Clinical and psychosocial outcomes of borderline personality disorder in childhood and adolescence: a systematic review. Psychol Med 45(11):2237–2251, 2015 25800970

Winsper C, Hall J, Strauss VY, et al: Aetiological pathways to borderline personality disorder symptoms in early adolescence: childhood dysregulated behaviour, maladaptive parenting and bully victimisation. Borderline Personal Disord Emot Dysregul 4:10, 2017 28588894

Winsper C, Wolke D, Scott J, et al: Psychopathological outcomes of adolescent borderline personality disorder symptoms. Aust N Z J Psychiatry 54(3):308–317, 2020 31647321

Wnuk S, McMain S, Links PS, et al: Factors related to dropout from treatment in two outpatient treatments for borderline personality disorder. J Pers Disord 27(6):716–726, 2013 23718760

Wolke D, Schreier A, Zanarini MC, et al: Bullied by peers in childhood and borderline personality symptoms at 11 years of age: a prospective study. J Child Psychol Psychiatry 53(8):846–855, 2012 22380520

Wong J, Bahji A, Khalid-Khan S: Psychotherapies for adolescents with subclinical and borderline personality disorder: a systematic review and meta-analysis. Can J Psychiatry 65(1):5–15, 2020 31558033

Wood JJ, Lynne-Landsman SD, Langer DA, et al: School attendance problems and youth psychopathology: structural cross-lagged regression models in three longitudinal data sets. Child Dev 83(1):351–366, 2012 22188462

World Health Organization: International Statistical Classification of Diseases and Related Health Problems, 11th Edition. Geneva, Switzerland, World Health Organization, 2019

Wright AGC, Zalewski M, Hallquist MN, et al: Developmental trajectories of borderline personality disorder symptoms and psychosocial functioning in adolescence. J Pers Disord 30(3):351–372, 2016a 26067158

Wright AG, Hopwood CJ, Skodol AE, Morey LC: Longitudinal validation of general and specific structural features of personality pathology. J Abnorm Psychol 125(8):1120–1134, 2016b 27819472

Yen S, Gagnon K, Spirito A: Borderline personality disorder in suicidal adolescents. Personal Ment Health 7(2):89–101, 2013 24343935

Yen S, Fuller AK, Solomon J, et al: Follow-up treatment utilization by hospitalized suicidal adolescents. J Psychiatr Pract 20(5):353–362, 2014 25226196

Zanarini MC: The Childhood Interview for DSM-IV Borderline Personality Disorder (CI-BPD). Belmont, MA, McLean Hospital and Harvard Medical School, 2003

Zanarini MC, Frankenburg FR: A preliminary, randomized trial of psychoeducation for women with borderline personality disorder. J Pers Disord 22(3):284–290, 2008 18540800

Zanarini MC, Gunderson JG, Frankenburg FR, et al: Discriminating borderline personality disorder from other axis II disorders. Am J Psychiatry 147(2):161–167, 1990 2301653

Zanarini MC, Frankenburg FR, Khera GS, et al: Treatment histories of borderline inpatients. Compr Psychiatry 42(2):144–150, 2001 11244151

Zanarini MC, Vujanovic AA, Parachini EA, et al: A screening measure for BPD: the McLean Screening Instrument for Borderline Personality Disorder (MSI-BPD). J Pers Disord 17(6):568–573, 2003 14744082

Zanarini MC, Frankenburg FR, Hennen J, et al: Axis I comorbidity in patients with borderline personality disorder: 6-year follow-up and prediction of time to remission. Am J Psychiatry 161(11):2108–2114, 2004 15514413

Zanarini MC, Frankenburg FR, Ridolfi ME, et al: Reported childhood onset of self-mutilation among borderline patients. J Pers Disord 20(1):9–15, 2006 16563075

Zanarini MC, Jacoby RJ, Frankenburg FR, et al: The 10-year course of social security disability income reported by patients with borderline personality disorder and axis II comparison subjects. J Pers Disord 23(4):346–356, 2009 19663655

Zanarini MC, Frankenburg FR, Reich DB, et al: Time-to-attainment of recovery from borderline personality disorder and its stability: a 10-year prospective follow-up study. Am J Psychiatry 167(6):663–667, 2010 20395399

Zanarini MC, Horwood J, Wolke D, et al: Prevalence of DSM-IV borderline personality disorder in two community samples: 6,330 English 11-year-olds and 34,653 American adults. J Pers Disord 25(5):607–619, 2011 22023298

Zanarini MC, Frankenburg FR, Reich DB, et al: Attainment and stability of sustained symptomatic remission and recovery among borderline patients and axis II comparison subjects: a 16-year prospective follow-up study. Am J Psychiatry 169(5):476–483, 2012 22737693

Zanarini MC, Conkey LC, Temes CM, et al: Randomized controlled trial of web-based psychoeducation for women with borderline personality disorder. J Clin Psychiatry 79(3):52–59, 2018 28703950

Zetterqvist M: The DSM-5 diagnosis of nonsuicidal self-injury disorder: a review of the empirical literature. Child Adolesc Psychiatry Ment Health 9:31, 2015 26417387

Zimmermann R, Fürer L, Schenk N, et al: Silence in the psychotherapy of adolescents with borderline personality pathology. Personal Disord April 23, 2020 Epub ahead of print 32324008

Appendix A

Relation of Good Psychiatric Management for Adolescents to Other Evidence-Based Treatments for Adolescent Borderline Personality Disorder

Cognitive Analytic Therapy Plus Helping Young People Early

Cognitive analytic therapy (CAT) is an individual psychotherapy rooted in object relations theory and cognitive psychology, and Helping Young People Early (HYPE) is a team-based early intervention service model of care in Australia that emphasizes case management, psychoeducation, engagement of caretakers, activity groups, and managing comorbidities. CAT involves exploring problematic internalized relational patterns and jointly formulating a clear developmental narrative about these patterns written in plain language and in diagram format. The focus is on developing more adaptive relational patterns.

Dialectical Behavior Therapy for Adolescents

Dialectical behavior therapy for adolescents (DBT-A) combines principles of cognitive-behavioral therapy (CBT) to promote change with Eastern mindfulness practices to promote acceptance. It includes individual sessions, multifamily skills group training, and family therapy and incorporates an adolescent-specific module ("Walking the Middle Path") that focuses on adolescent-family dialectical dilemmas such as dependence versus autonomy, leniency versus control, and pathologizing normative behaviors versus normalizing pathological behaviors. It teaches the patient how to regulate feelings and behaviors, with the therapist acting as a coach with extensive availability.

Emotion Regulation Training

Emotion regulation training (ERT) is based on Systems Training for Emotional Predictability and Problem Solving (STEPPS), a group-based treatment for adults with borderline personality disorder (BPD) that draws from CBT and incorporates DBT skills. It involves 17 group sessions that begin with psychoeducation and then teaches skills to promote self-awareness, individuality, and healthy lifestyle changes such as behavior modification plans, personal and mental health hygiene, eating, sleeping, and interpersonal relationships.

Mentalization-Based Treatment for Adolescents

Mentalization-Based Treatment for Adolescents (MBT-A) is an attachment-oriented, psychodynamically informed therapy that uses interventions from self-psychology and includes both individual and family therapy. The therapist adopts a "not-knowing" stance, monitoring levels of attachment activation while facilitating curiosity in patients to reappraise their own experiences and those of others (i.e., to mentalize). Its emphasis on thinking before reacting, even in states of high emotional arousal, is probably a process central to all effective therapies.

Transference-Focused Psychotherapy for Adolescents

Transference-focused psychotherapy for adolescents (TFP-A) is an individual psychotherapy approach founded in object relations psychoanalytic theory. It includes analysis of the roles and dynamics that develop in the treatment relationship, with interpretation of motives or feelings unknown to the patient. It retains a focus on the patient's experience of self and others in relationships as it develops in the treatment with the therapist (i.e., transference). Establishing a framework of expectations for the treatment at the outset assists in maintaining a stance of neutrality, where the therapist works to refrain from acting from a role reflecting split object relations (e.g., rescuer, protector, persecutor, harsh critic).

TABLE A–1. Comparative features of treatments

Therapy	Model	Intensity (hrs/wk)	Duration	Modalities	Focus	Managing S/SI
DBT-A	Emotional dysregulation	~3.6+	3–5 months	Individual, group (with family), family	Feelings and self-injurious behavior	Skills, phone coaching, extensive coverage
MBT-A	Misunderstood mental states	~1.25	1 year	Individual, family	Interpersonal, feelings, perspectives	Emergency department
TFP-A	Unintegrated self and other representations	~2	1 year	Individual, family	Interpersonal dynamics, affects	Emergency department
CAT + HYPE	Internalized maladaptive relationship patterns	~1–2	~6 months	Individual, medications, family, groups	Interpersonal and social	24/7 crisis team
ERT	Emotional dysregulation	~1.75	4.25 months	Group	Cognitions, feelings, behaviors	Emergency department

TABLE A–1. Comparative features of treatments (*continued*)

Therapy	Model	Intensity (hrs/wk)	Duration	Modalities	Focus	Managing S/SI
GPM-A	Interpersonal hypersensitivity	~1–2	As needed	Individual, medications, group, family	Interpersonal and social	Contingent, limited coverage

Note. CAT+HYPE=cognitive analytic therapy and helping young people early; DBT-A=dialectical behavior therapy for adolescents; ERT=emotion regulation training; GPM-A=good psychiatric management for adolescents; MBT-A=mentalization-based treatment for adolescents; S/SI=suicidality/suicidal ideation; TFP-A=transference-focused psychotherapy for adolescents.

Source. Adapted from Gunderson and Links 2014, p. 146.

TABLE A–2.   Research on comparative efficacy of treatments

Reference	Groups	Study design	Inclusion criteria	Sample characteristics (age, diagnosis)	Intervention
Cognitive analytic therapy					
Chanen et al. 2008a, 2009	CAT=41 Control=37 Historical control=32	RCT, based in Helping Young People Early clinic (for 15–18 year olds) specialized for BPD	Age 15–18; at least 3 DSM-IV criteria for BPD; at least 1 childhood risk factor; referred from the community; no psychotic illness	Mean age 17 years, 81% female, mean number of DSM criteria met 4.5	CAT: median of 13 CAT sessions. Also available to both CAT and control groups: pharmacotherapy, activity groups, crisis teams

TABLE A–2. Research on comparative efficacy of treatments (*continued*)

Comparison condition	Outcome variables	Duration, measurement points, and statistical model	Findings	Follow-up time and findings
Cognitive analytic therapy: Chanen et al. 2008a, 2009 (*continued*)				
Standardized GCC: a modular package controlling for availability, accessibility, and duration of care using a problem-solving model with modules for co-occurring problems; median of 11 sessions Historical TAU	SCID-II, YSR, semistructured parasuicidal behavior interview, SOFAS	43-week treatment, assessed at 6, 12, and 24 months; mixed-effects regression models	Both groups show significant positive effects, CAT faster on externalizing. Both CAT and GCC were superior to historical TAU.	Up to 24 months from baseline: CAT yields the greatest median improvement, but effect sizes are small; biggest effect on externalizing. CAT was superior to historical TAU on internalizing and on externalizing at 24 months. GCC was superior to TAU on internalizing and parasuicide.

TABLE A–2. Research on comparative efficacy of treatments *(continued)*

Reference	Groups	Study design	Inclusion criteria	Sample characteristics (age, diagnosis)	Intervention
Dialectical behavior therapy					
Cooney et al. 2010, 2012	DBT=14 Control=15	RCT, 6 months of DBT vs. uncontrolled TAU, in a naturalistic setting	Age 13–19; history of suicide attempt or self-injury in previous 3 months; one responsible caregiver	Mean age 16 years, 76% female, mean number of self-harm acts=6	DBT, individual therapy (weekly) and multifamily group skills training (110 minutes)

TABLE A–2. **Research on comparative efficacy of treatments** *(continued)*

Comparison condition	Outcome variables	Duration, measurement points, and statistical model	Findings	Follow-up time and findings
Dialectical behavior therapy: Cooney et al. 2010, 2012 (continued)				
TAU (including CBT, motivational interviewing focused on substance abuse, narrative-oriented family therapy)	SASII, RFL-A, BSSI	6-month treatment, baseline and posttreatment assessment, nonparametric models	Fewer people in TAU attempted suicide, but there was no difference in self-harm, emergency department visits, or substance use.	

TABLE A–2. Research on comparative efficacy of treatments *(continued)*

Reference	Groups	Study design	Inclusion criteria	Sample characteristics (age, diagnosis)	Intervention
Dialectical behavior therapy *(continued)*					
McCauley et al. 2018	DBT=72 IGST=65	RCT comparing DBT with IGST for reducing suicide attempts, NSSI, and self-harm in high risk youth recruited through emergency department, inpatient, outpatient, and community programs	At least 1 lifetime suicide attempt, elevated past-month suicidal ideation (≥24 on the SIQ-JR), self-injury repetition (≥3 lifetime self-harm episodes, including 1 in the prior 12 weeks), 3 or more BPD criteria	Mean age 14.9 years, 94.8% female	DBT: 6 months, weekly individual therapy, multifamily group skills training, youth and parent telephone coaching, and weekly therapist team consultation. Parents seen individually in session 1 and offered 7 or more family sessions

TABLE A–2. **Research on comparative efficacy of treatments** *(continued)*

Comparison condition	Outcome variables	Duration, measurement points, and statistical model	Findings	Follow-up time and findings
Dialectical behavior therapy, McCauley et al. 2018 *(continued)*				
IGST: 6 months, individual sessions, adolescent supportive group therapy, as-needed parent sessions (≤7 sessions), and weekly therapist team consultation	Suicide attempts, NSSI, self-harm (SASII), suicidal ideation (SIQ-JR)	6-month treatment, assessments at baseline and 3, 6, 9, and 12 months, mixed-model analysis of variance, nonlinear and hierarchical linear models	Significant advantages were found for DBT on all primary outcomes after treatment (suicide attempts, NSSI, self-harm). Treatment completion rates were higher for DBT than for IGST, but pattern-mixture models indicated that this difference did not informatively affect outcomes.	Rates of self-harm decreased through 1-year follow-up. The advantage of DBT decreased, with no statistically significant between-group differences from 6 to 12 months.

TABLE A–2. Research on comparative efficacy of treatments (continued)

Reference	Groups	Study design	Inclusion criteria	Sample characteristics (age, diagnosis)	Intervention
Dialectical behavior therapy (continued)					
Mehlum et al. 2014, 2019	DBT=39 EUC=38	RCT comparing DBT with EUC based in a metropolitan community psychiatric clinic, referred for current self-harm	Age 12–18; history of at least 2 episodes of self-harm (≥1 within the past 16 weeks); at least 2 DSM-IV BPD criteria (plus the self-destructive criterion) or at least 1 DSM-IV BPD criterion plus at least 2 subthreshold level criteria	Mean age 16 years, 88% female	Treatment: 19 weeks of DBT, 14 individual therapy sessions, 11 skills training group sessions, 3 family sessions

TABLE A–2. **Research on comparative efficacy of treatments** (*continued*)

Comparison condition	Outcome variables	Duration, measurement points, and statistical model	Findings	Follow-up time and findings
Dialectical behavior therapy: Mehlum et al., 2014, 2019 (*continued*)				
11 individual sessions, 6 family sessions, 1 group session	LPC, Short MFQ, BHS, MADRS, SIQ-JR	19-week treatment, assessments at 8, 15, and 19 weeks, mixed-effect multiple regression	Significant drop in self-harm in DBT but not in EUC. Differences emerged in the last third of the trial period. DBT had greater benefits on borderline symptoms and depression.	3-year follow-up: DBT-A remained superior in reducing self-harm. A substantial proportion (70.8%) of the effect of DBT on self-harm frequency over the long-term was mediated through a reduction in hopelessness during the trial phase. More than 3 months follow-up treatment after the trial was associated with further enhanced outcomes in DBT.

TABLE A–2.   Research on comparative efficacy of treatments (*continued*)

Reference	Groups	Study design	Inclusion criteria	Sample characteristics (age, diagnosis)	Intervention
Dialectical behavior therapy (*continued*)					
Rathus and Miller 2002	DBT=29 Control=82	Quasi-experimental study of consecutive admissions; patients were selected for DBT if they had a recent suicide attempt and 3 or more BPD criteria compared with other admissions	Suicide attempt in the past 16 weeks; diagnosis of BPD by SCID-II	Mean age 16.1 years (DBT) vs. 15 years (control); 93% (DBT) vs. 73% (control) female; 88% of the DBT group had BPD vs. 6% of the comparison group	DBT: 12 weeks, twice weekly, including parents in the skills training group and also in some individual therapy sessions

TABLE A–2.   Research on comparative efficacy of treatments (*continued*)

Comparison condition	Outcome variables	Duration, measurement points, and statistical model	Findings	Follow-up time and findings
Dialectical behavior therapy: Rathus and Miller 2002 (*continued*)				
TAU: 12 weeks; twice weekly individual and family sessions, supportive psychodynamic therapy	HASS, BDI, LPI, BSSI	12-week intervention, assessed at baseline and posttreatment, chi-square and other univariate statistics	Fewer hospital admissions in DBT condition but no difference in suicide attempts. More participants in DBT group completed treatment (62% vs. 40%).	

TABLE A–2. Research on comparative efficacy of treatments *(continued)*

Reference	Groups	Study design	Inclusion criteria	Sample characteristics (age, diagnosis)	Intervention
Mentalization-based treatment					
Bo et al. 2017	$N=34$ in group-based MBT	Group-based MBT in 3 outpatient clinics	Age 15–18; at least 4 DSM-5 BPD criteria; parents' or parent substitutes' commitment to participate in the MBT-Parents program	Mean age 16.4 years, 100% female	1-year program including 2 two individual case-formulation sessions (1 hour), 6 group-based MBT-I sessions (1.5 hours), then 34 sessions of MBT group therapy (1.5 hours)

TABLE A–2. **Research on comparative efficacy of treatments (*continued*)**

Comparison condition	Outcome variables	Duration, measurement points, and statistical model	Findings	Follow-up time and findings
Mentalization-based treatment: Bo et al. 2017 (*continued*)				
None	BPFS-C, YSR, BDI-Y, Risk-Taking and Self-Harm Inventory for Adolescents, Inventory of Parent and Peer Attachment-Revised, Reflective Function Questionnaire for Youth	12-month intervention, assessed at baseline and 12 months; paired sample t-tests to evaluate within-person change from baseline to end of treatment; assessment of clinically meaningful change	Significant reduction of BPFS-C score (84.5 to 64.6). Significant improvements for the general psychopathology, mentalizing, peer and parent attachment, self-harm, and depressive features. No significant improvements for externalizing psychopathology and risk-taking behavior. Clinically significant change for borderline pathology, mentalizing, peer trust, and parent trust.	

TABLE A–2. Research on comparative efficacy of treatments *(continued)*

Reference	Groups	Study design	Inclusion criteria	Sample characteristics (age, diagnosis)	Intervention
Mentalization-based treatment *(continued)*					
Rossouw and Fonagy 2012	MBT-A=40 Control=40	RCT of MBT-A or TAU, based in three community clinics; consecutive referrals of young people who self-harm	Age 12–17; at least 1 episode of self-harm within the past month; referred from the community because of history of intentional self-harm; no psychotic disorder	Mean age 15 years, 85% female, 97% depressed; 73% met criteria for BPD	MBT-A: individual session once per week plus family session once a month

TABLE A–2. **Research on comparative efficacy of treatments** *(continued)*

Comparison condition	Outcome variables	Duration, measurement points, and statistical model	Findings	Follow-up time and findings
Mentalization-based treatment: Rossouw and Fonagy 2012 *(continued)*				
NICE recommended evidence-based interventions (treatment as usual)	RTSHI, CI-BPD, MFQ, BPFS-C	12-month intervention, assessed at 3, 6, 9, and 12 months, mixed-effects regression and logistic regression models	Significant decrease in the mean number of self-harm attempts ($d=0.3$) and number self-harming at 9–12 months (56% vs. 82%); significant improvement in depression. At 12 months, 58% of TAU group and only 33% of MBT-A group met criteria for BPD.	

TABLE A–2. Research on comparative efficacy of treatments (*continued*)

Reference	Groups	Study design	Inclusion criteria	Sample characteristics (age, diagnosis)	Intervention
Mentalization-based treatment (continued)					
Laurenssen et al. 2014	MBT-A=11 No control group	Pilot study of MBT-A, independent of the treatment developers, based in one mental health center offering specialized inpatient treatment for adolescent personality disorders; referrals to the center	Age 14–18; at least 2 DSM-IV BPD criteria; no psychotic or organic brain disorder	Mean age 16.5 years, 100% female	MBT-A: 4 group sessions plus 1 individual session per week and 1 weekly session each of art therapy, writing therapy, and mentalizing cognitive therapy; psychiatric consultation, social work, and psychosocial coaching also available

TABLE A–2. Research on comparative efficacy of treatments (*continued*)

Comparison condition	Outcome variables	Duration, measurement points, and statistical model	Findings	Follow-up time and findings
Mentalization-based treatment: Laurenssen et al. 2014 (*continued*)				
None	BSI, SIPP-118, EuroQol EQ-5D	12-month intervention, assessed at baseline and 12 months; paired-samples t-tests	Significant decrease in symptomatic distress ($P<0.001$, $d=1.46$); marked improvements in personality functioning; significant improvement in quality of life ($P<0.05$, $d=1.11$); 91% showed reliable change and 18% moved to normal functioning	

TABLE A–2. Research on comparative efficacy of treatments *(continued)*

Reference	Groups	Study design	Inclusion criteria	Sample characteristics (age, diagnosis)	Intervention
Emotion regulation training					
Schuppert et al. 2009	ERT=23 Control=20	RCT based in five mental health centers; feasibility study testing randomization of young people with BPD symptoms to ERT+TAU or TAU alone	Age 14–19; at least 2 DSM-IV BPD criteria (mood instability plus ≥1 of impulsivity, recurrent suicidality/ self-harm, or anger)	Mean age 16 years, 88% female	17 weekly sessions (each 105 minutes) of ERT, group-based self-control CBT psychoeducation, plus TAU

TABLE A–2. Research on comparative efficacy of treatments *(continued)*

Comparison condition	Outcome variables	Duration, measurement points, and statistical model	Findings	Follow-up time and findings
Emotion regulation training: Schuppert et al. 2009 (continued)				
TAU: medication, individual psychotherapy, systemic therapy, psychiatric care tailored to individual need	MERLC, YSR	17 weeks, baseline and posttreatment, repeated measures ANOVA	No additional benefit from ERT. Internal locus of control increased with ERT. More subjects in ERT were lost to follow-up than in TAU.	

TABLE A–2. Research on comparative efficacy of treatments (continued)

Reference	Groups	Study design	Inclusion criteria	Sample characteristics (age, diagnosis)	Intervention
Emotion regulation training (continued)					
Schuppert et al. 2012	ERT=54 Control=55	RCT testing addition of ERT to TAU, based in five mental health centers; consecutive referrals for self-harm and other BPD symptoms	Age 14–19; at least 2 DSM-IV BPD criteria; score of 15 or more on total scale BPDSI	Mean age 16 years, 96% female; 73% met BPD criteria, 63% depressed	17 weekly sessions (each 105 minutes) of ERT, group-based self-control CBT psychoeducation

TABLE A–2.   Research on comparative efficacy of treatments (*continued*)

Comparison condition	Outcome variables	Duration, measurement points, and statistical model	Findings	Follow-up time and findings
Emotion regulation training: Schuppert et al. 2012 (*continued*)				
TAU (medication, individual CBT)	SCID-II, K-SADS, BPDSI, SCL90-R, Youth Quality of Life–Research Version; LPI; MERLC	6-month treatment; baseline, posttreatment and 12 months follow-up; mixed-effects models	Symptoms decreased regardless of treatment condition, no subgroup benefits specifically, low attrition	Improvements maintained at 6 months

TABLE A–2. **Research on comparative efficacy of treatments** *(continued)*

Note. ANOVA=analysis of variance; BDI=Beck Depression Inventory; BDI-Y=Beck Depression Inventory for Youth; BHS=Beck Hopelessness Scale; BPD=borderline personality disorder; BPDSI=Borderline Personality Disorder Severity Index; BPFS-C=Borderline Personality Features Scale for Children; BSI=Brief Symptom Inventory; BSL=Borderline Symptom List; BSSI=Beck Scale for Suicide Ideation; CAT=cognitive analytic therapy; CBT=cognitive-behavioral therapy; CI-BPD=Childhood Interview for Borderline Personality Disorder; DBT=dialectical behavior therapy; DSM=*Diagnostic and Statistical Manual of Mental Disorders*; ERT=emotion regulation training; EUC=enhanced usual care; EuroQol EQ-5D=European Quality of Life Scale; GCC=Good Clinical Care; HASS=Harkavy-Asnis Suicide Survey; IGST=individual and group supportive therapy; K-SADS=Kiddie Schedule for Affective Disorders and Schizophrenia; LPC=Lifetime Parasuicide Count; LPI=Life Problems Inventory; MADRS=Montgomery–Asberg Depression Rating Scale; MBT=mentalization-based treatment; MBT-A=MBT for adolescents; MBT-I=MBT-Introductory group; MERLC=Multidimensional Emotion Regulation Locus-of-control; MFQ=Mood and Feelings Questionnaire; NICE=National Institute for Clinical Excellence (U.K.); NSSI=nonsuicidal self-injury; RCT=randomized controlled trial; RFL-A=Reasons For Living Inventory for Adolescents; RTSHI=Risk-Taking and Self-Harm Inventory; SASII=Suicide Attempt-Self-Injury Interview; SCID-II=Structured Clinical Interview for DSM-IV Axis II Personality Disorders; SCL90-R=Symptom Checklist 90-Revised; SIPP-118=Severity Indices of Personality Problems; SIQ-JR=Suicidal Ideation Questionnaire Junior; SOFAS=Social and Occupational Functioning Assessment Scale; TAU=treatment as usual; YSR=Youth Self Report.

Source. Adapted from Sharp C, Kerr S, Chanen A: "Prevention and early identification of personality pathology: an AMPD informed model of clinical staging," in *Textbook of Personality Disorders*, 3rd Edition. Edited by Skodol A, Oldham J. Washington, DC, American Psychiatric Publishing, 2021, pp. 278–280. Copyright © 2021 American Psychiatric Association Publishing. Used with permission.

References

Bo S, Sharp C, Beck E, et al: First empirical evaluation of outcomes for mentalization-based group therapy for adolescents with BPD. Personal Disord 8(4):396–401, 2017 27845526

Chanen AM, Jackson HJ, McCutcheon LK, et al: Early intervention for adolescents with borderline personality disorder using cognitive analytic therapy: randomised controlled trial. Br J Psychiatry 193(6):477–484, 2008a 19043151

Chanen AM, McCutcheon LK, Germano D, et al: The HYPE Clinic: an early intervention service for borderline personality disorder. J Psychiatr Pract 15(3):163–172, 2009 19461389

Cooney EB, Davis KL, Thompson P, et al: Feasibility of evaluating DBT for self-harming adolescents: a small randomised controlled trial. Auckland, Te Pou o Te Whakaaro Nui, New Zealand Mental Health Research, August 2010. Available at: www.tepou.co.nz/uploads/files/resource-assets/feasibility-of-evaluating-dbt-for-self-harming-adolescents.pdf. Accessed September 15, 2020.

Cooney E, Davis K, Thompson P, et al: Feasibility of comparing dialectical behavior therapy with treatment as usual for suicidal and self-injuring adolescents: follow-up data from a small randomized controlled trial, in Is DBT Effective With Multi-Problem Adolescents? Show Me the Data! An International Presentation of Three Randomized Trials Evaluating DBT With Adolescents. Miller AL (Chair). Symposium conducted at the Annual Meeting of the Association of Behavioral and Cognitive Therapies, National Harbor, MD, November 15–18, 2012

Gunderson JG, Links P: Handbook of Good Psychiatric Management for Borderline Personality Disorder. Washington, DC, American Psychiatric Publishing, 2014

Laurenssen EM, Hutsebaut J, Feenstra DJ, et al: Feasibility of mentalization-based treatment for adolescents with borderline symptoms: a pilot study. Psychotherapy (Chic) 51(1):159–166, 2014 24059741

McCauley E, Berk MS, Asarnow JR, et al: Efficacy of dialectical behavior therapy for adolescents at high risk for suicide: a randomized clinical trial. JAMA Psychiatry 75(8):777–785, 2018 29926087

Mehlum L, Tørmoen AJ, Ramberg M, et al: Dialectical behavior therapy for adolescents with repeated suicidal and self-harming behavior: a randomized trial. J Am Acad Child Adolesc Psychiatry 53(10):1082–1091, 2014 25245352

Mehlum L, Ramleth RK, Tørmoen AJ, et al: Long term effectiveness of dialectical behavior therapy versus enhanced usual care for adolescents with self-harming and suicidal behavior. J Child Psychol Psychiatry 60(10):1112–1122, 2019 31127612

Rathus JH, Miller AL: Dialectical behavior therapy adapted for suicidal adolescents. Suicide Life Threat Behav 32(2):146–157, 2002 12079031

Rossouw TI, Fonagy P: Mentalization-based treatment for self-harm in adolescents: a randomized controlled trial. J Am Acad Child Adolesc Psychiatry 51(12):1304–1313, 2012 23200287

Schuppert HM, Giesen-Bloo J, van Gemert TG, et al: Effectiveness of an emotion regulation group training for adolescents—a randomized controlled pilot study. Clin Psychol Psychother 16(6):467–478, 2009 19630069

Schuppert HM, Timmerman ME, Bloo J, et al: Emotion regulation training for adolescents with borderline personality disorder traits: a randomized controlled trial. J Am Acad Child Adolesc Psychiatry 51(12):1314–1323, 2012 23200288

Appendix B

General Psychiatric Management Adherence Scale

THE GENERAL PSYCHIATRIC MANAGEMENT Adherence Scale (GPMAS; Kolla et al. 2009) assesses the adherence of delivered interventions to good psychiatric management (GPM) treatment. Clinicians are asked to score the amount of emphasis placed during the previous therapy session on each of 48 items, from 1 (no emphasis) to 5 (major emphasis). The scale is scored by computing the overall mean score as well as subscale scores. In a trial of 10-session GPM (Kolly et al. 2016), adherence to GPM as measured by the GPMAS explained 23% of the decrease in BPD symptoms and 16% of the improvement in general symptoms of patients with BPD. This scale can be used to assess adherence and also as a guide or checklist for keeping track of what to do and what not to do.

	1 **Not at all**	**2**	**3**	**4**	**5** **Completely** **present**

Subscale 1: Assessment procedures

1. Completing safety evaluation
2. Determining treatment setting or level of care required
3. Assessing for presence of comorbid disorders
4. Assessing functional impairments, needs, and goals
5. Examining intrapsychic conflicts and defenses
6. Examining development progress and arrests
7. Examining adaptive and maladaptive coping styles
8. Examining psychosocial stressors
9. Examining strengths
10. Determining other concurrent treatments needed

Subscale 2: Establishing treatment contract

11. Establishing the treatment framework
12. Determining readiness for psychotherapy
13. Encouraging concurrent treatments

	1 Not at all	2	3	4	5 Completely present

Subscale 2: Establishing treatment contract *(continued)*

14. Identifying ongoing care providers

15. Developing crisis management plan

Subscale 3: Ongoing case management

16. Responding to crises and safety monitoring

17. Establishing a therapeutic framework and alliance

18. Maintaining a therapeutic framework and alliance

19. Providing education about the disorder and its treatment

20. Coordinating the treatment effort

21. Monitoring and reassessing clinical status and treatment plan

22. Encouraging multi-modal treatment

23. Intervening regarding functioning

Subscale 4: General principles of psychotherapy

24. Some form of psychotherapy offered

25. Demonstrating flexibility

26. Attending to role of patient preference in terms of the focus of the psychotherapy

	1 Not at all	2	3	4	5 Completely present

Subscale 4: General principles of psychotherapy *(continued)*

27. Dealing with setting boundaries

28. Conducting skills training

29. Demonstrating empathy and validation

30. Conveying feasible expectations

31. Set up expectations for responsible behavior

32. Let positive transference alone

33. Active with early signs of negative transference

Subscale 5: Focus on feelings

34. Focusing on identification of feelings

35. Commenting about facial expressions

36. Remarking on body language

37. Clarifying maladaptive responses to feelings

38. Connecting behaviors to events or thoughts or feelings

39. Inquiring whether anything new has been learned

40. Fostering clients' interest or curiosity

	1 Not at all	2	3	4	5 Completely present

Subscale 5: Focus on feelings *(continued)*

41. Using clients' words and language

Subscale 6: Specific therapeutic issues

42. Taking a rehabilitation focus

43. Expanding the focus away from self-harm

44. Visiting early trauma in session

45. Exploring body image distortion

46. Expecting or encouraging competitiveness

47. Discussing intersession contacts

48. Discussing termination

Source. Adapted from Kolla et al. 2009.

References

Kolla NJ, Links PS, McMain S, et al: Demonstrating adherence to guidelines for the treatment of patients with borderline personality disorder. Can J Psychiatry 54(3):181–189, 2009 19321022

Kolly S, Despland JN, de Roten Y, et al: Therapist adherence to good psychiatric practice in a short-term treatment for borderline personality disorder. J Nerv Ment Dis 204(7):489–493, 2016 21787770

Appendix C

Online Good Psychiatric Management Training

McLean Gunderson Personality Disorders Institute's Online Course on Good Psychiatric Management

- Website: http://hms.harvard.edu/BPD

Good psychiatric management (GPM; formerly general psychiatric management) has been demonstrated to match the effectiveness of dialectical behavior therapy in treating patients with borderline personality disorder (BPD; McMain et al. 2009). The 8-hour McLean Gunderson Personality Disorders Institute course teaches mental health professionals what they need to know to become competent providers who can derive satisfaction from treating these patients.

Through lectures, case vignettes, and interactive decision points, the course covers management strategies such as practicality, good sense, and flexibility. It describes techniques and interventions that facilitate the patient's trust and willingness to become a proactive collaborator. It reviews guidelines for managing the common and usually most burdensome issues of managing suicidality and self-harm (e.g., intersession crises, threats as a call for help, excessive use of emergency departments or hospitals). Furthermore, it describes how and when psychiatrists can usefully integrate group, family, or other psychotherapies.

Date: Available until July 13, 2022
Cost: $25
Provided by: Harvard Medical School Continuing Medical Education; Gunderson Personality Disorders Institute at McLean Hospital
Length: 8 hours

Source.   Adapted from Choi-Kain and Gunderson 2019.

References

Choi-Kain LW, Gunderson JG (eds): Applications of Good Psychiatric Management for Borderline Personality Disorder. Washington, DC, American Psychiatric Association Publishing, 2019

McMain SF, Links PS, Gnam WH, et al: A randomized trial of dialectical behavior therapy versus general psychiatric management for borderline personality disorder. Am J Psychiatry 166(12):1365–1374, 2009 19755574

Appendix D

Guidelines for Families

Setting Goals: Go Slowly

- Remember that change is difficult to achieve and fraught with fears. Be cautious about suggesting that "great" progress has been made or giving "You can do it" reassurances. Progress evokes fears of abandonment.

The families of people with borderline personality disorder (BPD) can tell countless stories of instances in which their son or daughter went into crisis just as that person was beginning to function better or to take on more responsibility. The coupling of improvement with a relapse is confusing and frustrating but has a logic to it. When people make progress—by working, leaving day treatment, helping in the home, diminishing self-destructive behaviors, or living alone—they are becoming more independent. They run the risk that those around them who have been supportive, concerned, and protective will pull away, concluding that their work is done. The supplies of emotional and financial assistance may soon dry up, leaving these individuals to fend for themselves in the world. Thus, they fear abandonment. Their response to the fear is a relapse. They may not make a conscious decision to relapse, but fear and anxiety can drive them to use old coping methods. Missed days at work; self-mutilation; a suicide attempt; or a bout of overeating, purging, or drinking may be a sign that lets everyone around know that the individual remains in distress and needs their help. Such relapses may compel people around them to take responsibility for them through protective measures such as hospitalization. Once hospitalized, the individual has returned to his or her most regressed state in which he or she has no responsibilities while others take care of him or her.

When signs of progress appear, family members can reduce the risk of relapse by not showing too much excitement about the progress and by cautioning the individual to move slowly. This is why experienced members of the hospital staff tell patients with BPD during discharge not that they feel confident about their prospects, but that they know the patient will confront many hard problems ahead. It is important to acknowledge progress with a pat on the back, but at the same time it is also necessary to convey understanding that progress is very difficult to achieve. It does not mean that the person has overcome his or her emotional struggles. You can do this by avoiding statements such as "You've made great progress" or "I'm so impressed with the change in you." Such messages imply that you think the person is well or over his or her prior problems. Even statements of reassurance such as "That wasn't so hard" or "I knew you could do it" suggest that you are minimizing their struggle. A message such as the following can be more empathic and less risky: "Your progress shows real effort. You've worked hard. I'm pleased that you were able to do it, but I'm worried that this is all too stressful for you."

- Lower your expectations. Set realistic goals that are attainable. Solve big problems in small steps. Work on one thing at a time. "Big," long-term goals lead to discouragement and failure.

Although individuals with BPD may have many obvious strengths such as intelligence, ambition, good looks, and artistic talent, they nonetheless are disadvantaged by severe emotional vulnerabilities as they set about making use of those talents. Usually, people with BPD and their family members have aspirations based on these strengths. Patients or their family may push for return to college, graduate school, or a training program that will prepare the young person for financial independence. Family members may wish to have the patient move into his or her own apartment and care for himself or herself more independently. Fueled by such high ambitions, the person with BPD will take a large step forward at a time. He or she may insist on returning to college full time despite undergoing recent hospitalizations, for example. Of course, such grand plans do not consider the individual's handicaps of affect dyscontrol, black-and-white thinking, and intolerance of aloneness. Affect dyscontrol may mean that, for example, receiving a B on the first exam could lead to an inappropriate display of anger if the person thinks the grade is unfair, to a self-destructive act if the person feels he or she is a total failure, or severe anxiety if the person believes that success in school would lead to decreased parental concern. The overriding issue about success in the vocational arena is the threat of independence—much desired but fraught with fear of abandonment. The result of too large a step forward all at once is often a crashing swing in the opposite direction, like the swing of a pendulum. The person often relapses to a regressed state and may even require hospitalization.

A major task for families is to slow down the pace at which they or the patient seek to achieve goals. By slowing down, they prevent the sharp swings of the pendulum as described and prevent experiences of failure that are blows to the individual's self-confidence. By lowering expectations and setting small goals to be achieved step by step, patients and families have greater chances of success without relapse. Goals must be realistic. For example, an individual who left college midsemester after becoming depressed and suicidal under the pressure most likely could not return to college full time a few months later and expect success. A more realistic goal is for that person to try one course at a time while he or she is stabilizing. Goals must be achieved in small steps. Individuals with BPD who have always lived with their parents might not be able to move straight from their parents' home. The plan can be broken down into smaller steps in which the individual first moves to a halfway house and then into a supervised apartment. Only after he or she has achieved some stability in those settings should the individual take the major step of living alone.

Not only should goals be broken down into steps, but they should be taken on one step at a time. For example, if the patient and the family have goals for both the completion of school and independent living, it may be wisest to work on only one of the two goals at a time.

Managing the Family Environment

- Keep things cool and calm. Appreciation is normal. Tone it down. Disagreement is normal. Tone it down, too.

This guideline is a reminder of the central message of our educational program: The person with BPD is handicapped in his ability to tolerate stress in relationships (i.e., rejection, criticism, disagreements) and can, therefore, benefit from a cool, calm home environment. It is vital to keep in mind the extent to which people with BPD struggle emotionally each day. Although their internal experience can be difficult to convey, we explain it by summarizing three areas of difficulty: affect dyscontrol, intolerance of aloneness, and black-and-white thinking.

- **Affect dyscontrol:** A person with BPD has feelings that dramatically fluctuate in the course of each day and that are particularly intense. These emotions, or affects, often hit hard. We have all experienced such intense feelings at times. Take, for example, the sensation of pounding heart and dread that you may feel when you suddenly realize that you have made a mistake at work that might be very costly or embarrassing to your business. The person with BPD feels such intense emotion on a regular basis. Most people can soothe themselves through such emotional experiences by telling themselves that they will find a way to compensate for the mistake or reminding themselves that it is only human to make mistakes. People with BPD lack that ability to soothe themselves. An example can also be drawn from family conflict. We have all had moments in which we feel rage toward the people we love. We typically calm ourselves in such situations by devising a plan for having a heart-to-heart talk with the family member or by deciding to let things blow over. Individuals with BPD feel such rage in its full intensity and without being able to soothe themselves through the use of coping strategies. This results in an inappropriate expression of hostility or in acting out of feelings (e.g., drinking, cutting).
- **Intolerance of aloneness:** A person with BPD typically feels desperate at the prospect of any separation—a family member's or therapist's vacation, breakup of a romance, departure of a friend. Most of us would probably miss the absent family member, therapist, or friend, but people with BPD typically feel intense panic. They are unable to conjure up images of the absent person to soothe themselves. They cannot tell themselves, "That person really cares about me and will be back again to help me." Their memory fails them, and they feel soothed and cared for by the other person only when that person is present. Thus, the other person's absence is experienced as abandonment. Individuals with BPD may even keep these painful thoughts and feelings out of mind by using a defense mechanism called dissociation, which consists of a bizarre and disturbing feeling of being unreal or separate from one's body.
- **Black-and-white thinking (dichotomous thinking):** Along with extremes of emotion come extremes in thinking. People with BPD tend to have extreme opinions. Others are often experienced as being either all good or all bad. When the other person is caring and supportive, the person with BPD views him or her as a savior, someone endowed with special qualities. When the other person fails, disagrees, or disapproves in some way, the person with BPD views him or her as being evil and uncaring. The handicap is in the inability to view other people more realistically, as mixtures of good and bad qualities.

This review of the handicaps of people with BPD is a reminder that they have a significantly impaired ability to tolerate stress. Therefore, the family members can help them achieve stability by creating a cool, calm home environment. This means slowing down and taking a deep breath when crises arise rather than reacting with great emotion. It means setting smaller goals for the person with BPD so as to diminish the pressure he or she is experiencing. It means communicating when you are calm and in a manner that is calm. It does not mean sweeping disappointments and disagreements under the rug by avoiding discussion of them. It does mean that conflict needs to be addressed in a cool but direct manner without use of put-downs. Subsequent guidelines will provide methods for communicating in this fashion.

- Maintain family routines as much as possible. Stay in touch with family and friends. There is more to life than problems, so don't give up the good times.

Often, when a member of the family has a severe mental illness, everyone in the family can become isolated as a result. The handling of the problems can absorb much time and energy. People often stay away from friends to hide a problem they feel as stigmatizing and shameful. The result of this isolation can be only anger and tension. Everyone needs friends, parties, and vacations to relax and unwind. By making a point of having good times, everyone can cool down and approach life's problems with improved perspective. The home environment will naturally be cooler. You should have good times not only for your own sake but for the sake of the whole family.

- Find time to talk. Chats about light or neutral matters are helpful. Schedule times for this if you need to.

Too often, when family members are in conflict with one another or are burdened by the management of severe emotional problems, they forget to take time out to talk about matters other than illness. Such discussions are valuable for many reasons. People with BPD often devote all their time and energy to their illness by going to multiple therapies each week, by attending day treatment, and so on. The result is that they miss opportunities to explore and use their variety of talents and interests. Their sense of self is typically weak and may be weakened further by this total focus on problems and the attention devoted to their being ill. When family members take time to talk about matters unrelated to illness, they encourage and acknowledge the healthier aspects of the person's identity and the development of new interests. Such discussions also lighten the tension between family members by introducing some humor and distraction. Thus, they help you to follow the guideline to keep things cool and calm.

Managing Crisis: Pay Attention but Stay Calm

- Don't get defensive in the face of accusations and criticisms. However unfair, say little and don't fight. Allow yourself to be hurt. Admit to whatever is true in the criticisms.

When people who love each other get angry at each other, they may hurl heavy insults in a fit of rage. This is especially true for people with BPD because they tend to feel a great deal of anger. The natural response to criticism that feels unfair is to defend oneself. However, as anyone who has ever tried to defend oneself in such a situation knows, defending yourself doesn't work. A person who is enraged is not able to think through an alternative perspective in a cool, rational fashion. Attempts to defend oneself only fuel the fire. Essentially, defensiveness suggests that you believe the other person's anger is unwarranted, a message that leads to greater rage. Given that individuals who are expressing rage with words are not posing threat of physical danger to themselves or others, it is wisest to simply listen without arguing.

What that individual wants most is to be heard. Of course, listening without arguing means getting hurt because it is very painful to recognize that someone you love could feel so wronged by you. Sometimes the accusations hurt because they seem to be so frankly false and unfair. Other times, they may hurt because they contain some kernel of truth. If you feel that there is some truth in what you're hearing, admit it with a statement such as "I think you're on to something. I can see that I've hurt you and I'm sorry."

Remember that such anger is part of the problem for people with BPD. It may be that they were born with a very aggressive nature. The anger may represent one side of their feelings, which can rapidly reverse. (See earlier discussion of black-and-white thinking.) Keeping these points in mind can help you to avoid taking the anger personally.

Some families never talk in this way, and to do so may seem unnatural and uncomfortable at first. There may be a hundred reasons why there is no opportunity for such communication, but families need to make the time. The time can be scheduled in advance and posted on the refrigerator door. For example, everyone may agree to eat dinner together a few times a week, with an agreement that there will be no discussions of problems and conflict at these times. Eventually, the discussions can become habit and scheduling will no longer be necessary.

- Self-destructive acts or threats require attention. Don't ignore them. Don't panic. It's good to know about them. Do not keep secrets about such acts or threats. Talk about them openly with your family member and make sure professionals know about them.

There are many ways in which people with BPD and their family members may see trouble approaching. Threats and hints of self-destructiveness may include a variety of provocative behaviors. Individuals with BPD may speak of wanting to kill themselves. They may become isolative. They may superficially scratch themselves. Some parents have noticed that their children shave their head and color their hair neon at times when they are in distress. More commonly, what will be evident is not eating or reckless behavior. Sometimes the evidence is blunt, such as a suicide gesture made in the parent's presence. Trouble may be anticipated when separations or vacations occur.

When families see the signs of trouble, they may be reluctant to address them. Sometimes, adolescents with BPD insist that their family "butt out." They may appeal to their right to privacy. Other times, family members dread speaking directly about a problem because the discussion may be difficult. They may fear that they will cause a problem where there might not be one by "putting ideas into someone's head." In fact, families fear for their child's safety in these situations because they know their children well and know the warning signs of trouble from experience. Problems are not created by asking questions. By addressing provocative behaviors and triggers in advance, family members can help to avert further trouble. People with BPD often have difficulty talking about their feelings and instead tend to act on them in destructive ways. Therefore, addressing a problem openly by inquiring with the adolescent or speaking to his or her therapist helps the person with BPD to deal with his or her feelings using words rather than actions.

Privacy is, of course, a great concern when you are dealing with an adult. However, in these situations the competing value of impending danger is safety. When making difficult decisions about whether to call your loved one's therapist about a concern or to call an ambulance, you must weight concern for safety against concern for privacy. Most people would agree that safety comes first. There may be a temptation to under-react in order to protect the individual's privacy. At the same time, there may be a temptation to overreact in ways that give the person reinforcement for his or her behavior. One young woman with BPD told her mother excitedly during an ambulance ride to a psychiatric hospital, "I've never been in an ambulance before!" Families must apply judgment to their individual situation. Therapists can be helpful in anticipating crises and establishing plans that fit the individual family's needs.

- Listen. People need to have their negative feelings heard. Don't say, "It isn't so." Don't try to make the feelings go away. Using words to express fear, loneliness, inadequacy, anger, or needs is good. It's better to use words than to act out on feelings.

When feelings are expressed openly, they can be painful to hear. A daughter may tell her parents that she feels abandoned or unloved by them. A parent may tell his child that he's at the end of his rope with frustration. Listening is the best way to help an emotional person to cool off. People appreciate being heard and having their feelings acknowledged. This does not mean that you have to agree. Let's look at the methods for listening. One method is to remain silent while looking interested and concerned. You may ask some questions to convey your interest. For example, you might ask, "How long have you felt this way?" or "What happened that triggered your feelings?" Notice that these gestures and questions imply interest but not agreement. Another method of listening is to make statements expressing what you believe you have heard. With these statements, you prove that you are actually hearing what the other person is saying. For example, if your daughter tells you she feels like you don't love her, you can say, even as you are contemplating how ridiculous that belief is, "You feel like I don't love you?!?" When a child is telling her parents that she feels as if she has been treated unfairly by them, parents may respond, "You feel cheated, huh?" Notice once again, these empathic statements do not imply agreement.

Do not rush to argue with your family member about his or her feelings or talk him or her out of those feelings. As stated previously, such arguing can be fruitless and frustrating to the person who wants to be heard. Remember, even when it may feel difficult to acknowledge feelings that you believe have no basis in reality, it pays to reward such expression. It is good for people, especially individuals with BPD, to put their feelings into words, no matter how much those feelings are based on distortions. If people find the verbal expression of their feelings to be rewarding, they are less likely to act out on feelings in destructive ways.

Feelings of being lonely, different, and inadequate need to be heard. By hearing your family member and demonstrating that you have heard him or her using the methods described above, you help the individual to feel a little less lonely and isolated. Such feelings are a common, everyday experience for people with BPD. Parents usually do not know and often do not want to believe that their child feels these ways. The feelings become a bit less painful once they are shared.

Family members may be quick to try to talk someone out of such feelings by arguing and denying the feelings. Such arguments are quite frustrating and disappointing to the person expressing the feelings. If the feelings are denied when they are expressed verbally, the individual may need to act on them in order to get his or her message across.

Addressing Problems: Collaborate and Be Consistent

- When solving a family member's problems, *always* involve the family member in identifying what needs to be done; ask whether the person can "do" what's needed in the solution; ask whether he or she wants you to help him or her "do" what's needed.

Problems are best tackled through open discussion in the family. Everyone needs to be part of the discussion. People are most likely to do their part when they are asked for their participation and their views about the solution are respected. It is important to ask each family member whether he or she feels able to do the steps called for in the planned solution.

By asking, you show recognition of how difficult the task may be for the other person. This goes hand in hand with acknowledging the difficulty of changing. You may feel a powerful urge to step in and help another family member. Your help may be appreciated or may be an unwanted intrusion. By asking if your help is wanted before you step in, you make sure that your assistance is less likely to be resented.

- Family members need to act in concert with one another. Parental inconsistencies fuel severe family conflicts. Develop strategies that everyone can stick to.

Family members may have sharply contrasting views about how to handle any given problem behavior in their relative with BPD. When they each act on their different views, they undo the effect of each other's efforts. The typical result is increasing tension and resentment between family members as well as lack of progress in overcoming the problem.

An example will illustrate the point: Renee frequently calls home asking for financial bailouts. She has developed a large credit card debt. She wants new clothing. She has been unable to save enough money to pay her rent. Despite her constant desire for funds, she is unable to take financial responsibility by holding down a job or living on a budget. Her father expresses a stern attitude, refusing to provide the funds, and with each request he insists that Renee take responsibility for working out the problem herself. Her mother meanwhile softens easily with each request and gives Renee the funds she wants. She feels that providing the extra financial help is a way of easing her daughter's emotional stress. The father then resents the mother's undoing of his efforts at limit setting, while the mother finds the father to be excessively harsh and blames him for Renee's worsening course. Renee's behavior persists, of course, because there is no cohesive plan for dealing with the financial issue that both parents can stick to. With some communication, they can develop a plan that provides an appropriate amount of financial support, one that would not be viewed as too harsh by the mother, but would not be considered excessively generous in the father's eyes. Renee will adhere to the plan only after both parents adhere to it.

Brothers and sisters can also become involved in these family conflicts and interfere with each other's efforts in handling problems. In these situations, family members need to communicate more openly about their contrasting views on a problem, hear each other's perspectives, and then develop a plan that everyone can stick to.

- If you have concerns about medications or therapist interventions, make sure that both the person with BPD and his or her therapist, doctor, and/or treatment team know. If you have financial responsibility, you have the right to address your concerns to the therapist or doctor.

Families may have a variety of concerns about their loved one's medication usage. They may wonder whether the psychiatrist is aware of the side effects the patient is experiencing. Can the psychiatrist see how sedated or obese the individual has become? Is he or she subjecting the patient to danger by prescribing too many medications? Families and friends may wonder if the doctor or therapist knows the extent of the patient's noncompliance or history of substance abuse.

When family members have such concerns, they often feel that they should not interfere, or they are told by the patient not to interfere. However, if family members play a major supportive role in the patient's life, such as providing financial or emotional support, or by sharing their home, they should make efforts to participate in treatment planning for him or her. They can play that role by contacting the doctor or therapist directly themselves to express their concerns. Therapists cannot release information about patients who are older than 18 years without consent, but they can hear and learn from the reports of the patient's close family and friends. Sometimes they will work with family members or friends, but obviously with the patient's consent.

Limit Setting: Be Direct but Careful

- Set limits by stating the limits of your tolerance. Let your expectations be known in clear, simple language. Everyone needs to know what is expected of them.

Expectations need to be set forth in a clear manner. Too often, people assume that the members of their family should know their expectations automatically. It is often useful to give up such assumptions.

The best way to express an expectation is to avoid attaching any threats. For example, you might say, "I want you to take a shower at least every other day." When expressed in that fashion, the statement puts responsibility on the other person to fulfill the expectation. Often in these situations, family members are tempted to enforce an expectation by attaching threats: "If you don't take a shower at least every other day, I will ask you to move out." The first problem with that statement is that the person making the statement is taking on the responsibility. He or she is saying, "*I* will take action if *you* do not fulfill your responsibility" as opposed to giving the message "*You* need to take responsibility." The second problem with that statement is that the person making it may not really intend to carry out the threat if pushed. The threat becomes an empty expression of hostility. Of course, there may come a point at which family members feel compelled to give an ultimatum with the true intention to act on it. We discuss this situation later.

- Do not protect family members from the natural consequences of their actions. Allow them to learn about reality. Bumping into a few walls is usually necessary.

People with BPD can engage in dangerous, harmful, and costly behaviors. The emotional and financial toll to the individual and the family can be tremendous. Nonetheless, family members may sometimes go to great lengths to give in to the individual's wishes, undo the damage, or protect everyone from embarrassment. The results of these protective ways are complex. First and foremost, the troublesome behavior is likely to persist because it has cost no price or has brought the individual some kind of reward. Second, the family members are likely to become enraged because they resent having sacrificed integrity, money, and good will in their efforts to be protective. In this case, tensions in the home mount even though the hope of instigating the protective measures was to prevent tension. Meanwhile, the anger may be rewarding on some level to the individual because it makes him or her the focus of attention, even if that attention is negative. Third, the individual may begin to show these behaviors outside the family and face greater harm and loss in the real world than he or she would have faced in the family setting. Thus, the attempt to protect leaves the individual unprepared for the real world. Some examples will illustrate the point.

- Chloe, a 16-year-old girl, stuffs a handful of pills in her mouth in the presence of her mother, Diane. Diane puts her hand into Chloe's mouth to sweep out the pills. It is reasonable to prevent medical harm in this way. Diane then considers calling an ambulance because she can see that Chloe is suicidal and at risk of harming herself. However, this option would have some very negative consequences. Chloe and the family would face the embarrassment of having an ambulance in front of the house. Chloe does not wish to go to the hospital and would become enraged and out of control if Diane calls for an ambulance. In this situation, Diane might be strongly tempted not to call the ambulance in order to avoid her daughter's wrath and to preserve the family's image in the neighborhood. She might rationalize the decision by convincing herself that Chloe is not in fact in immediate danger. The primary problem with that choice is that it keeps Chloe from attaining much needed help at a point when she has been and could still be suicidal. Diane would be aiding Chloe in denial of the problem. Medical expertise is needed to determine whether Chloe is at risk of harming herself. If her dramatic gesture is not given sufficient attention, she likely would escalate. As she escalates, she may make an even more dramatic gesture and face greater physical harm. Furthermore, if an ambulance is not called for fear of incurring her wrath, Chloe would receive the message that she can control others by threatening to become enraged.

- Ashley, a 25-year-old woman, steals money from her family members while she is living with them. The family members express great anger at her and sometimes threaten to ask her to move out, but they never take any real action. When she asks to borrow money, they give her a loan despite the fact that she never pays back such loans. They fear that if they do not lend the money, she may steal it from someone outside the family, thus leading to legal trouble for her and humiliation for everyone else involved. In this case, the family has taught Ashley that she can get away with stealing. She has essentially blackmailed them. They give her what she wants because they are living in fear. Ashley's behavior is very likely to persist as long as no limits are set on it. The family could cease to protect her by insisting that she move out or by stopping the loans. If she does steal from someone outside the family and faces legal consequences, this may prove to be a valuable lesson about reality. Legal consequences may influence her to change and subsequently function better outside the family.

- Sara, a 20-year old woman who has had multiple psychiatric hospitalizations recently and has been unable to hold down any employment, decides that she wants to return to college full time. She asks her parents to help pay her tuition. The parents, who watch their daughter spend most of her day in bed, are skeptical that she will be able to remain in school for an entire semester and pass her courses. The tuition payments represent great financial hardship for them. Nonetheless, they agree to support the plan because they do not want to believe Sara is as dysfunctional as she behaves and because they know she will become enraged if they do not. With this action, they have given Sara a dangerous "You can do it" message. Furthermore, they have demonstrated to her that displays of anger can control her parents' choices. A more realistic plan would be for Sara to take one course at a time to prove that she can do it and then return to school full time only after she has demonstrated the ability to maintain such a commitment despite her emotional troubles. In this plan, she faces a natural consequence for her recent low functioning. The plan calls on her to take responsibility in order to obtain a privilege she desires.

Each of the cases illustrates the hazards of being protective when a loved one is making unwise choices or engaging in frankly dangerous behavior. By setting limits on these choices and behaviors, family members can motivate individuals to take on greater responsibility and have appropriate limits within themselves. The decision to set limits is often the hardest decision for family members to make. It involves watching a loved one struggle with frustration and anger. It is important for parents to remember that their job is not to spare their children these feelings but to teach them to live with those feelings as all people need to do.

- Do not tolerate abusive treatment such as tantrums, threats, hitting, and spitting. Walk away and return to discuss the issue later.

Frank tantrums are not tolerable. There is a range of ways to set limits on them. A mild gesture would be to walk out of the room to avoid rewarding the tantrum with attention. A more aggressive gesture would be to call an ambulance. Many families fear taking the latter step because they do not want an ambulance in front of their home or because they do not want to incur the wrath of the person having the tantrum. When torn by such feelings, you must consider the opposing issues. Safety may be a concern when someone is violent and out of control. Most people would agree that safety takes priority over privacy. Furthermore, by neglecting to get proper medical attention for out-of-control behavior, you are turning a silent ear to it, which only leads to further escalation. The acting out is a cry for help. If a cry for help is not heard, it only becomes louder.

- Be cautious about using threats and ultimatums. They are a last resort. Do not use threats and ultimatums as a means of convincing others to change. Give them only when you can and will carry through. Let others—including professionals—help you decide when to give them.

When one family member can no longer tolerate another member's behavior, he or she may reach the point of giving an ultimatum. This means threatening to take action if the other person does not cooperate. For example, when a daughter will not take a shower or get out of bed much of the day, an exasperated parent may want to tell her that she will have to move out if she does not change her ways. The parent may hope that fear will push her to change. At the same time, the parent may not be serious about the threat. When the daughter continues to refuse to cooperate, the parent may back down, proving that the threat was an empty one. When ultimatums are used in this way, they become useless, except to produce some hostility. Thus, you should give ultimatums only when you seriously intend to act on them. In order to be serious about the ultimatum, the person giving it probably has to be at the point where he or she feels unable to live with the other person's behavior.

Source. Adapted from Gunderson J, Berkowitz C: Family Guidelines: Multiple Family Group Program at McLean Hospital. 2020. New England Personality Disorder Association, 2020.
Available at: www.borderlinepersonalitydisorder.org/family connections/ family guidelines/. Accessed July 21, 2020.

Appendix E

Online Psychoeducation Resources

All resources are adapted from Choi-Kain and Gunderson 2019.

General Resources for Consumers, Families, and Clinicians

National Education Alliance for Borderline Personality Disorder (NEABPD)

www.borderlinepersonalitydisorder.com

Information: provides information about BPD for patients, families, Family Connections leaders, and professionals; also includes information on the Global Alliance for Prevention and Early Intervention for BPD (GAP) and a podcast. The Family Guidelines are provided in various languages.

Links to national organizations, research, and treatment

Referral source: none; has a "Looking for Treatment" page with suggestions on finding the right treatment and professional

Lists: recommendations of publications, books, a library of articles, and the NEABPD journal; a media library, including conference presentation and course/workshop videos

McLean Hospital Borderline Personality Disorder Family and Consumer Education

www.mcleanhospital.org/borderline-personality-disorder-patient-and-family-education-initiative

Initiative: webinar series by BPD experts at McLean Hospital

Videos for all audiences: webinars include (but are not limited to) Common Questions About Borderline Personality Disorder and What You Can Do to Help; How Can I Recognize Borderline Personality Disorder? (conducted in Spanish); Difficult Conversations: How to Discuss Borderline Personality Disorder With a Loved One; General Psychiatric Management (GPM) for the Treatment of Borderline Personality Disorder; Family Struggles and Strategies to Address Common Challenges; Symptoms of Borderline Personality Disorder in Adolescents

Project Air

www.projectairstrategy.org

Fact sheets: provides resources relevant to the patient, families, schools, and clinicians. For patients, answer useful and relevant questions such as "You've been diagnosed with BPD; what now?" Offers relatable useful facts, self-help resources, and parenting tools. For clinicians, offers basic toolkit of pragmatic guidance.

Adolescent Brief Intervention Manual for Complex Mental Health Issues: brief (four session) intervention centered on creating a care plan for the young person and a support plan for his or her carer. May be useful as a stepping stone before longer-term care.

Borderline Personality Disorder Support Services in South Australia

http://bpdsa.com.au

Website: provides information for consumers, carers, and clinicians. For consumers and carers, there are several links to helpful websites such as Project Air and SANE Australia. There are also resources for finding care for individuals living in Australia. For clinicians, there are links to relevant research, websites, and some in-person and online training options.

Online library: provides a link to a free online library of research and resources regarding how clinicians can best work with families and carers. The contents of the library include videos, training manuals, and empirical research articles.

Treatment and Research Advancements for Borderline Personality Disorder (TARA4BPD)

www.tara4bpd.org

About BPD: information on the disorder, common comorbidities, suicide, and research

Treatment: information on treatment, with sections covering dialectical behavior therapy and mentalization-based treatment

Family help: information on the TARA method—a training to help families learn how to support themselves and the individual with BPD, taught in virtual workshops

Help for BPD sufferers: information on a monthly psychoeducation meeting in New York and some metaphor-based tips (e.g., carrying a stone, the self-oiling machine)

Help for clinicians: opportunity to join a referral list by entering contact information and qualifications

Finding help: contact information for TARA, information on research studies, and recommended readings

BPD Foundation

www.bpdfoundation.org.au

Website: psychoeducational materials on BPD, coexisting disorders, and treatments, including books, presentations and conferences, and research articles

Lists: online resources for people with BPD, their carers, and general practitioners

Provides additional resources on help tips, recovery, and multicultural mental health

Resources for Consumers and Their Families

National Alliance on Mental Illness (NAMI)

www.nami.org

Information: information on BPD under the topic "About Mental Illness" (click on "Mental Health Conditions" and then "Borderline Personality Disorder"). Provides information about etiology, comorbidities, treatment, self-harm, and medications

Links: information on treatment modalities for BPD, "A BPD Brief" (Gunderson and Berkowitz 2006a), substance use disorders, self-injury, family connection reading list, and mental illness discussion groups and a link to the NEABPD and National Institute of Mental Health (NIMH) websites

Referral source: state and local affiliates that provide support, education, information, referral, and advocacy

Emotions Matter

https://emotionsmatterbpd.org

What is BPD? Factual information on prevalence, BPD (e.g., neurobiology, symptoms), common misconceptions, and treatment

Programs: online peer support groups, social connections, Facebook group, advocacy efforts

Resources: list of organizations, online resources, and books and access to downloadable guides for students with BPD and those affected by self-harm for the student, the carers, and school administrators

Personality Disorder Awareness Network (PDAN)

www.pdan.org

Information: provides information on personality disorders, including BPD, a blog, online parenting programs, and recordings of past webinars

Links to national and international organizations such as NAMI, NIMH, and the Australian Organization for BPD

Referral source: links to Theravive, a network of mental health professionals in the United States and Canada; GoodTherapy.org; and PsychologyToday.com

Lists: recommended books such as helpful options for children (e.g., *The Weather House: Living with a Parent with Borderline Personality Disorder*)

New York Presbyterian BPD Resource Center

www.nyp.org/bpdresourcecenter

Information: provides information on diagnosis and treatment; instructional videos by experts regarding symptoms, treatment, and recovery; and audio recordings of individuals with BPD telling their own stories

Lists: informational websites, recommended books by both experts and individuals with BPD, and publications for professionals

SANE Australia: Guide to Borderline Personality Disorder

www.sane.org/information-stories/facts-and-guides/borderline-personality-disorder#help-for-people-with-bpd

Help for people with BPD: walks the individual with BPD through what a BPD diagnosis means, options for care, staying safe in a crisis, and getting support

Help for family, friends, and carers: provides a guide for families and friends regarding how to connect with a person with BPD, how to look out for themselves, and how to help someone in a crisis

Reference

Choi-Kain LW, Gunderson JG (eds): Applications of Good Psychiatric Management for Borderline Personality Disorder. Washington, DC, American Psychiatric Association Publishing, 2019

Index

Page numbers printed in **boldface** type refer to tables and figures.